Vocal Rehabilitation

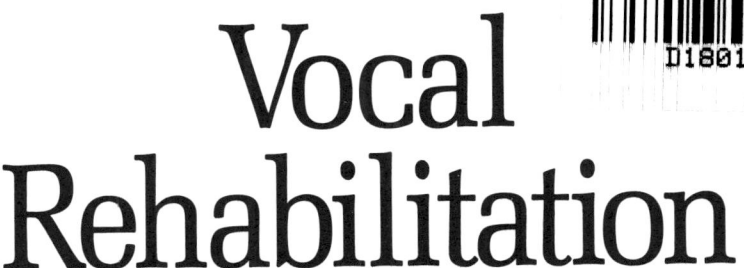

D1801788

A PRACTICE
BOOK FOR VOICE
IMPROVEMENT

THIRD EDITION

VIRGINIA L. AGNELLO
CINDY GARCIA

pro·ed

8700 Shoal Creek Boulevard
Austin, Texas 78757

Virginia L. Agnello is a speech pathologist
who specializes in the voice and its disorders.
Cindy Garcia is a fiction and technical writer.

© 1990 by PRO-ED, Inc.

Previously published under the title *A Workbook for Voice Improvement*,
©1983, 1977 by PRO-ED, Inc.

Printed in the United States of America

Library of Congress Cataloging-in-Publication Data

Agnello, Virginia L.
    Vocal rehabilitation: a practice book for voice improvement /
Virginia L. Agnello, Cindy Garcia. — 3rd ed.
        p. cm.
    Rev. ed. of: A workbook for voice improvement. 2nd ed. c1983.
    ISBN 0-89079-233-X
    1. Voice culture — Exercises. I. Garcia, Cindy. II. Agnello,
Virginia L. Workbook for voice improvement. III. Title.
RF540.A38   1990
616.85'506 — dc20   90-8336
                                                                    CIP

pro·ed
8700 Shoal Creek Boulevard
Austin, Texas 78757

10   9   8   7   6   5   4   3   95

Contents

Contents • **v**

Preface

The person who has a clear, effective, and artistic speaking voice and who has come by this voice naturally has been given a most unique gift. However, many people find that their voices are not serving them as they desire and that they are not functioning as effectively as they wish, in either their professions or private lives. In these cases the voice is probably not being used correctly, therefore not reaching its full potential.

The voice is an instrument; we need to go through certain steps in order to master it. One rule in developing new vocal skills is that practice really does make perfect; however, practice of any kind is not always exciting. As a speech and voice pathologist I have been asked many times by my patients, "Do you know of a book that would help me at home with my practice?" They have also remarked, "I find it difficult to practice because it's so monotonous and boring." For these reasons I designed this practice book for vocal rehabilitation so that it can be used by either the speech pathologist or the patient working at home.

I have made efforts to incorporate a sprinkling of philosophy and enough drama and humor to stimulate the interest of both the patient and the clinician.

I feel deep gratitude to Morton Cooper, PhD, for the training I received under his guidance and for the opportunity of working with so many stimulating people.

I want to give thanks also to my co-author, Cindy Garcia, who had the discipline necessary to write special sentences and paragraphs according to a formula that was new to her.

Most of all, my particular thanks to my patients, because without them this practice book would not have been possible.

Virginia L. Agnello

Acknowledgments

We wish to express our sincere appreciation to the following publishers and individuals who have granted permission to reproduce certain poems, excerpts, and selections used in this book.

William F. Boni for "A Prospectus for the Remodeled Chewing Gum Corporation" by Will Rogers in *Reading to Others*, edited by Argus Tresidder, copyright 1940. Published by Scott, Foresman and Company. Reprinted with the permission of William F. Boni.

Morton Cooper, PhD, for the exercise "Me-Me One." Reprinted with the permission of Morton Cooper.

Doubleday & Company, Inc., for the excerpt from *The Ra Expeditions*, copyright 1971 by George Allen & Unwin, Ltd. Reprinted by permission of Doubleday & Company, Inc.

Farrar, Straus & Giroux, Inc., for the poem from *Kalahari* by Jens Bjerre, copyright 1958 by Carit Andersens Forlag and copyright 1960 by Michael Joseph Ltd. Reprinted with the permission of Farrar, Straus & Giroux, Inc.

Harcourt, Brace, Jovanovich, Inc., for the poem "Dance of the Animals" from *The African Saga* by Blaise Cendrars. Reprinted with the permission of Harcourt, Brace, Jovanovich, Inc.

Harper & Row Publishers, Inc., for the excerpt from *Captain Cousteau's Underwater Treasury* by Jacques-Yves Cousteau and James Dugan, copyright 1959. Reprinted with the permission of Harper & Row Publishers, Inc.

Harper & Row Publishers, Inc., for the excerpt from *Europe and Elsewhere* by Mark Twain. Reprinted with the permission of Harper & Row Publishers, Inc.

Houghton Mifflin Company for the excerpt from *The Hobbit* by J.R.R. Tolkien, copyright 1966 by J.R.R. Tolkien. Reprinted with the permission of Houghton Mifflin Company.

Liveright Publishing Corporation for the selection from "The Dybbuk" by A. Ansky (Solomon Rappoport), copyright 1926 by Henry G. Alsberg. Copyright renewed 1953 by Henry G. Alsberg and Winifred Katzin.

Macmillan Publishing Co., Inc., for the excerpt from *The Magician's Nephew* by C.S. Lewis, copyright 1955 by Macmillan Publishing Co., Inc. Reprinted with the permission of Macmillan Publishing Co., Inc.

Oxford University Press, Inc., for the selection from *Venus Observed: A Play* by Christopher Fry, copyright 1949 by Christopher Fry. Reprinted with the permission of Oxford University Press, Inc.

Pacific Telephone Company for the two selections "The Critic in Hiding" and "When the Swallows Come Back to Capistrano" from *California Vignettes*.

Peter Pauper Press for the selections from *Comic Epitaphs from the Very Best Old Graveyards*, copyright 1957 by the Peter Pauper Press.

Peter Pauper Press for the poems in *The Jade Flute*: "Seeing You Off" by Po Chu-i, "The Poet and the Flood" by Tu Fu, "Eternity" from *The Way of Virtue*, copyright 1960 by the Peter Pauper Press.

Prentice-Hall, Inc., for the selection "The American Case" by Ralph Linton, *The Study of Man: An Introduction*, copyright 1936, pp. 326–327. Reprinted by permission of Prentice-Hall, Inc.

The Viking Press for the excerpts from *My Family and Other Animals* by Gerald Durrell, copyright 1956 by Gerald M. Durrell. Reprinted by permission of the Viking Press.

The Viking Press for the two poems from *2-Rabbit 7-Wind: Poems of Ancient Mexico* by Toni de Gerez, copyright 1971 by Toni de Gerez. Reprinted by permission of the Viking Press.

Walker & Company, Inc., for the two poems from the book *A Crocodile Has Me by the Leg* by Leonard W. Doob, published by Walker & Company, Inc., copyright 1966 by Leonard W. Doob.

Every effort has been made to ascertain the ownership of the material chosen for this practice book in order to give credit to copyright holders. If any errors occur in our acknowledgments they were unintentional and will be corrected in subsequent editions as they are brought to our attention.

Introduction

When it was decided to put together a practice book for voice problems, it soon became evident that such a book could not incorporate all of the theories and techniques used today. Therefore, it should be noted that the framework for *Vocal Rehabilitation: A Practice Book for Voice Improvement* was developed solely from the experience of one speech pathologist who has had success working with voice cases. The philosophy this book goes by is the theory that certain characteristics contribute to an effective speaking voice — pitch, tone focus, volume, quality, and rate. They should be coordinated with breath support from the midsection or diaphragm. If a voice breaks down, the cause is usually misuse or abuse. It then stands to reason that one or more of the vocal characteristics is out of balance. My experience is that when a person learns to correctly coordinate the vocal variables and to carry that coordination over to his or her life-style, vocal rehabilitation is a success, and the person experiences the joy of a healthy, effective voice.

APPLICATIONS AND ORGANIZATION OF THE BOOK

The central goal of the exercises here is the development of a person's optimal pitch and correct tone focus. But for those clinicians whose treatment goals are different, the word lists and sentences may be adapted. In other words, the practice book is not a means of treatment, but merely a tool for vocal rehabilitation. It is not *the* way, it is only one of many.

The procedures outlined in this book work well with most patients regardless of whether their vocal folds are normal or show pathology. The speech pathologist can modify the exercises to suit the specific voice disorder. The goals are to eliminate vocal misuse or abuse and to gain a healthy, proficient voice.

Under no circumstances should this book be used without the guidance of a competent voice clinician; it is not for "do-it-yourselfers." Any benefit from these exercises is due to direction by the clinician.

We have made every effort to present this practice book in a simple form. Professional terms and phonetic symbols that might be unknown to the layman have been eliminated.

From the authors' point of view, midsection breathing is an integral part of developing a healthy voice. The science of breathing is based on a definite philosophy and, as such, needs a book of its own to describe and teach breathing from the midsection or diaphragm. References are made for the coordination of breathing with the other characteristics of voice throughout the exercises; the assumption is that this method of breathing is being taught as the patient progresses.

The book is divided into seven steps. These steps proceed from simple one-word exercises to sentences to paragraphs and longer readings that place greater demands upon the patient's vocal skill. Each step is preceded by a short explanation of the purpose of the exercises, along with their goals and procedures.

When appropriate, the optimal or natural pitch of the patient should be established by the clinician before starting the exercises found in this book. Once the optimal pitch has been established, it is of course necessary for the patient to be able to recognize and produce it without the help of the clinician; however, experience has proven that in order for the patient to use his optimal pitch as a lifestyle, it is helpful to practice all of the exercises in this book a note or so above the patient's optimal pitch level. Also, we have assumed that the clinician is modifying the other vocal variables of tone focus, quality, volume, and rate as needed during vocal rehabilitation.

Success or failure of vocal rehabilitation is determined by the skill and sensitivity of the clinician, regardless of the techniques used, since good interaction between clinician and patient is the key to successful treatment. It is hoped that the creative energies of both will join to make the practice of the following exercises a lively and productive experience.

A NOTE ABOUT PRACTICE

Practicing 5 minutes out of every hour throughout the day has been found to be the most productive. However, the life-styles of many people will not allow this. It is important, nevertheless, to be sure that the day is started with at least a few minutes of practice. This sets the tone for the day and often helps you to remember your voice throughout the day.

If it is not possible to practice the few minutes out of each hour, then you could budget time in the morning, afternoon, and evening, according to the schedule set up by you and your clinician. Short periods of practice sprinkled throughout the day seem to be more effective than one long session at night.

A cassette tape recorder can be a helpful tool. Your ear must be trained to detect the changes that are taking place throughout the process of voice change. The immediate feedback and objective listening made possible by a tape recorder is one way of accomplishing this.

It is also necessary to warm up before starting your practice or using your voice professionally, because in essence you are a "vocal athlete." Your clinician may choose the warm-up exercises thought to be best for you. When great demands have been put on the vocal instrument, cooling down is always advisable.

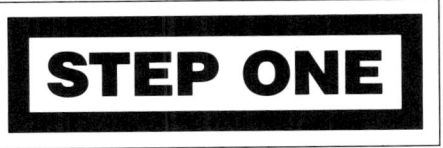

Basic Exercises

PURPOSE

This first exercise is one of the most important. The nasal sounds *m* and *n*, because of their nature, help to keep the pitch and tone focus in the mask of the face. The automatic function of counting helps you to keep your attention on your voice. Combining the nasal sounds with vowels and counting results in an exercise that can be practiced in many different situations, such as when you're driving or busy around the house. This exercise may be equated with the practice of scales on the piano. Just as the scales are needed for a pianist to strengthen his or her fingers to perform a concerto, the following exercise is needed to strengthen the muscles that are used to support your new pitch.

Although the final goal of vocal rehabilitation is to habituate the optimal pitch and correct tone focus among other vocal variables that may need changing, it has been observed that when the new voice is ready to be used in all spontaneous speaking situations, the pitch automatically drops a note or so. Therefore it is advised that this exercise and all those that follow be practiced slightly above the optimal pitch. This technique also aids in strengthening the musculature. Throughout the book the term "practice pitch" will be used to differentiate between the optimal pitch and the one used in practice.

It is wise to use the counting exercises at the beginning of each treatment session or practice at home. They are particularly good for warming up the voice before going on to more demanding vocal tasks.

GOAL To establish your practice pitch level and correct tone focus.

PROCEDURE

1. Utter spontaneously "hi" or "hello" as if you are delighted to see someone. This technique often helps you to find your practice pitch; however, your clinician will guide you in locating it. The numbers 1–10 are then added to the "hi" or "hello," for example, "hello-one," "hello-two," "hello-three," etc.

2. Practice the exercise "me-me one" in the same way as the "hello-one." This exercise may be practiced as if you are asking a question. For example, start with "hi" and then continue with "me-me one?" "me-me two?" etc. Maintain your practice pitch throughout the entire count of 10.

EXERCISES

1.   hello   1–10
            hi   1–10

2.*		
	me-me	1–10
	mo-mo	1–10
	moo-moo	1–10
	ma-ma	1–10
	may-may	1–10
	ne-ne	1–10
	no-no	1–10
	noo-noo	1–10
	na-na	1–10
	nay-nay	1–10
	nim-nim	1–10
	ze-ze	1–10
	zo-zo	1–10
	zoo-zoo	1–10
	za-za	1–10
	zay-zay	1–10
	zim-zim	1–10

3. You can practice the days of the week stressing the first syllable on your practice pitch. For example, MONday, TUESday, WEDNESday. Be careful not to drop the pitch of "day" too low.

4. Practice the months of the year and the alphabet in the same way.

---

* Copyright 1967, Morton Cooper, PhD.

STEP TWO

Word Lists

PURPOSE

The word lists in the following section have been chosen for the vowels and diphthongs within the stressed syllable. These vowels and diphthongs have been found to help you stay on your practice pitch. As you put forth the effort to maintain your practice pitch and to speak each word slowly, the exercise may seem somewhat singsongy or monotonous, but don't be concerned about the sound at this stage.

The lists of words are organized in the following way: The first column places the particular vowel or diphthong in the middle of the word. The second column stresses the sound at the end of the word, and in the third column it is found at the beginning of the word. This structure is chosen because, for some people, initiating a vowel sound is difficult. Your clinician will guide you from one list to another according to your individual rate of progress.

The Isolated Word List at the end of this section includes all of the consonant sounds and their blends. This list is included as a test to uncover any possible problem sounds.

GOAL To establish the practice pitch and correct tone focus on single words.

PROCEDURE

1. Spontaneously say "hi," "me-me," or "hello," whichever is easiest to use as an aid in locating your practice pitch. From now on these words will be called the carrier phrase.

2. Say the carrier phrase and 5 or 6 words. Repeat the carrier phrase and say 5 or 6 more words until you've completed each row on the page. For example: "Hi-bean, creak, cheese, etc." and then again, "Hi-deep, leave, grief, etc."

3. Make efforts to keep the carrier phrase and the words on the same pitch.

4. If you are lowering your pitch, your clinician will probably start you on words that stress the vowel $\bar{o}$ as in go, since the vowels $\bar{e}$ and $\overline{oo}$ have a tendency to help you raise your pitch rather than lower it. The exercise would then be "$\bar{o}$—bold, zone, broke, etc., $\bar{o}$—mean, joke, float, etc."

5. When you feel sure of your practice pitch, you may drop the carrier phrase and just say the words. Practice them slowly.

6. Try to keep the tone focus forward in the mask of the face. It often helps to think of projecting the voice forward onto an imaginary target. For example, you might imagine a bull's-eye on the wall in front of you, and your voice then becomes the arrow.

7. Add each new page of words under the guidance of your clinician.

8. The rate of progress is an individual thing, and it may be that the goal of this step is met before you have practiced the entire spectrum of words. If your clinician thinks you are developing skill in maintaining your correct pitch

and tone focus, you will be started on Step Three before finishing this one. These two steps are often integrated.

9. Go through the Isolated Word List in the same way as suggested above in number 2. Check for any sounds that seem difficult to produce clearly. If none are found, there is no need to continue practicing this step.

10. After each page in this section has been practiced, the word lists may then be chosen arbitrarily.

WORD LISTS

The vowel ē as in *even* is the sound to be stressed in the following words.

Middle	End	Beginning
bean	bee	each
creak	free	eel
cheese	flea	eke
deep	key	eaves
leave	glee	evil
grief	he	evening
geese	me	either
heel	knee	easel
steal	tree	even
peek	see	eaten
steed	plea	eagle
weep	she	Easter
speech	spree	eager
peace	three	Eden
feeble	tea	edict
fever	wee	Egypt
teacher	fee	easy
reason	gee	ego

WEBSTER: $\overline{oo}$
OTHER SPELLINGS: u, ou, ue, ew, o, ui

The vowel $\overline{oo}$ as in *moon* is the sound to be stressed in the following words.

Middle	End
boost	coo
juice	do
school	blue
ghoul	flew
plume	glue
dude	too
boom	true
spoof	rue
spool	slew
proof	shoe
rumor	shrew
movies	zoo
noodle	through
loony	who
brewing	grew
prudent	clue
super	brew
tuna	sue
ruby	voodoo

WEBSTER: ū
OTHER SPELLINGS: u, ou, ue, ew, o, ui

The vowel ū as in use is the sound to be stressed in the following words.

Middle	End	Beginning
cube	few	you
huge	cue	use
fume	new	union
mute	pew	usury
feud	chew	eulogy
cute	lieu	usual
mule	view	unify
pure	hue	unit
music	mew	unicorn
beauty	skew	youth
future	you	euphemism
humid	spew	ewer
fuse	adieu	eunuch
humor	debut	Utah
pupil	renew	Euclid
feudal	imbue	yule
human	review	useful
muse	argue	uniform

The vowel ô as in *off* is the sound to be stressed in the following words.

Middle	End	Beginning
cough	paw	all
moth	law	ought
broth	maw	audible
cause	jaw	awful
pause	caw	auto
fought	raw	almost
dog	claw	automat
paunch	squaw	aura
brought	craw	audit
laundry	flaw	auger
bog	straw	ostrich
haunt	draw	author
crawl	thaw	awkward
broad	slaw	often
maul	saw	August
wrong	gnaw	autumn
fraught	yaw	auction
song	foresaw	auburn
toss	macaw	also
frothy	withdraw	office

The diphthong ī as in *ice* is the sound to be stressed in the following words.

Middle	End	Beginning
five	cry	isle
slide	spy	ice
prime	die	I'm
knight	fry	I'd
pride	my	ivory
time	nigh	eyebrow
tide	sigh	isolated
rhyme	tie	icicle
thrice	pie	iris
Nile	sky	Irish
mine	try	idolize
trial	lie	item
spiral	buy	eyes
cycle	rye	iron
fight	sty	Iceland
mice	pry	Ireland
mighty	ply	island
white	sly	icon
riot	spry	idol
tribal	fly	iodine

The diphthong *ou* as in *out* is the sound to be stressed in the following words.

Middle	End	Beginning
mouth	prow	owl
flout	cow	out
gown	now	ours
scout	bough	ouch
crown	how	ounce
joust	chow	hour
vowel	wow	oust
pout	vow	outcast
stout	plow	outrage
flounce	brow	outlet
dowry	thou	outline
brown	scow	outright
sour	pow	outfit
flower	allow	
power	kowtow	
house	endow	
roust	avow	
shower	bow-wow	

WEBSTER: ō
OTHER SPELLINGS: oh, ow, ew, oa, oe

The diphthong ō as in *old* is the sound to be stressed in the following words.

Middle	End	Beginning
bold	dough	oak
moan	flow	oaf
broke	blow	old
joke	mow	ode
float	tow	only
ghost	bow	own
soul	no	oath
poke	foe	oboe
poem	hoe	okra
roam	sew	opus
dope	stow	open
zone	crow	odor
croak	show	ocean
hoax	slow	opal
coal	pro	omen
cope	low	oval
toad	glow	over
bowling	though	oleo

Note: This diphthong has been found to be one of the best sounds to develop the quality of the voice; it cannot be practiced too much.

WEBSTER: ā
OTHER SPELLINGS: ay, ai, ea, ey, ei

The diphthong ā as in *age* is the sound to be stressed in the following words.

Middle	End	Beginning
fate	neigh	eight
jail	bray	ache
dame	pray	ape
mane	ray	age
gale	say	ace
fame	gray	aid
break	play	angel
train	stray	able
chaste	spray	ailing
freight	sleigh	atheist
tape	tray	apron
frail	jay	acorn
brain	weigh	aviator
slain	they	aviary
danger	repay	amiable
daily	okay	ancient
daisy	portray	alien
neighbor	display	apex
failure	betray	April
radio	delay	acre

The diphthong *oi* as in *boy* is the sound to be stressed in the following words.

Middle	End	Beginning
foil	toy	oil
boil	boy	oink
toil	poi	oyster
coiled	coy	oilcloth
voice	joy	ointment
hoist	cloy	oily
coin	ploy	
spoil	troy	
join	soy	
loiter	enjoy	
doily	alloy	
moisten	destroy	
foible	employ	
broiled	ahoy	
poison	annoy	
boisterous	deploy	
void	decoy	
royal	convoy	
choice		
noise		

ISOLATED WORD LIST

The following words include all the sounds, plus the *l*, *r*, and *s* blends.

1. bank
   been
   book

2. cheer
   child
   chin

3. day
   dip
   done

4. face
   fact
   feel

5. gave
   get
   girl

6. had
   head
   heart

7. just
   jail
   jump

8. keep
   kind
   king

9. late
   learn
   light

10. blink
    blow
    blossom

11. clay
    clock
    clever

12. fly
    flash
    float

13. glad
    glory
    glimmer

14. play
    plumb
    please

15. slide
    slept
    slim

16. splash
    splinter
    splendor

17. maid
    might
    men

18. name
    next
    night

19. part
    pay
    point

20. queen
    quiet
    quilt

21. ring
    right
    room

22. bring
    broom
    brass

23. crowd
    crab
    cream

24. draw
    dry
    drink

25. friend
    frost
    fresh

26. great
    green
    grace

27. praise
    pride
    prince

28. try
    trick
    travel

29. three
    thrown
    thrill

30. shrink
    shrug
    shrine

31. serve
    said
    seen

32. sky
    skate
    scarlet

33. small
    smash
    smooth

34. snow
    snap
    sniff

35. spoon
    speak
    sparkle

36. star
    story
    stair

37. squeak
    squirrel
    squander

38. sweet
    swim
    swift

39. spring
    spread
    spree

40. scrub
    screen
    scroll

41. strong
    straw
    stream

42. she
    show
    shall

43. take
    tell
    ten

44. think
    thank
    thought

45. though
    there
    thee

46. vast
    view
    visit

47. warm
    wear
    west

48. where
    why
    white

49. year
    yet
    yard

50. zest
    zoo
    zebra

Sentences

PURPOSE

This next step in the process of vocal rehabilitation is meant to increase your vocal skills. As the word lists become easier for you, it is necessary to try connecting the words into sentences. You may discover it's more difficult to sustain a sentence using your practice pitch and correct tone focus than managing just one word. Each page of sentences in Section A emphasizes one particular vowel and/or diphthong and has been written to correlate with the lists in Step Two.

The material in Section B stresses no particular sound. These sentences are quotations chosen from many sources to add color and appeal to your practice.

GOAL To maintain your practice pitch and correct tone focus throughout a sentence.

PROCEDURE

Section A

1. Be sure to start on your practice pitch before speaking the sentence. Remember to always use "Hi" as a springboard into your practice pitch and to "think forward" in order to keep your tone focus in the mask of the face.

2. Your natural inclination may be to drop your pitch at the end of a sentence, but be careful not to drop it too low. Keep in mind that this is only an exercise, and a somewhat monotonous pitch is expected.

3. A good way to practice is first to warm up with the "me-me ones"; second, practice any word list you wish; and third, select the page of sentences that corresponds to the word list of your choice. In this way as you record and listen to the exercise, you have completed a 10- or 15-minute practice period.

Section B

As your vocal skills progress, you may note that maintaining your practice pitch and correct tone focus is becoming easier. When this takes place, begin to read the sentences for their meanings with natural inflection.

SECTION A—SENTENCES

These sentences stress the vowel ē as in *even*.

1. Our Siamese cat teased Mrs. Beasley's monkey, Frieda, who shrieked and scurried up our peach tree.

2. The three buddies went on a spree beginning in Miami Beach and ending in a Boston beanery.

3. Steve heard an eerie tune seeping through a hole behind the tapestry, but he fell asleep before he could investigate.

4. The gypsy's tiny feet scaled the steep ravine as if she were a young deer.

5. In the evenings Old Bundy told stories about his weasel, Sweet Godfrey, as mischievous a creature as ever breathed.

6. The Golden Fleece gleamed like the eastern sun as Jason carried it to Greece.

7. The police refused to believe that Aberdeen had been peeped at by travelers from Venus.

8. The tea leaves promised Irene a booming career in beekeeping and TV repair.

9. Maxine was sorry she got even by stealing Phoebe's pickles and replaced them with a steaming crock of Chinese peas.

10. The thief careened through the streets of Baghdad, pursued by angry mercenaries of the queen.

11. The hero of the TV series was a meek bird fancier, who solved everything from missing parakeets to stolen condors.

12. Aaron's portrait of the goddess Diana, seated with her fabled beasts about her, seems to speak of worlds we have long forgotten.

These sentences stress the vowel o͞o as in *moon*.

1. The gold doubloons lay buried in a bamboo grove at the edge of the island's voodoo country.

2. The cooling noodle drooped around Irwin's spoon, a pale and gloomy curlicue.

3. Boone concluded that the clever goose had loosened a group of slats before she flew the coop.

4. Rupert chewed the early morning fruit, which oozed with juice and April dew.

5. By Tuesday, Brute MacGoogle was the dirtiest shooter in the Yellow Coyote Saloon.

6. The trooper stopped to help Miss Mamie Purdue free her ankles from some rudely determined roots.

7. We thought Mrs. Dooley was fooling when she ran around crying "Boo!" — until one night she flew off on a two-dollar broom.

8. Old Blue snoozed in the shade while I threw my line into the soupy pool crooning to all those reclusive catfish.

9. Grandma spoke of an early doom if I kept my rendez-vous with young Hoot Riley on his orange Suzuki.

10. The poor guy tried to act aloof every time Julie walked past in her new bikini, but he kept spilling his prune sherbet.

11. I'll never forget Aunt Trudy singing "Chattanooga Choo Choo" wearing green satin and orange tulle.

12. As a cartoonist I started doodling in school, even though it was strictly taboo.

These sentences stress the vowel ū as in use.

1. Lionel the unicorn amused us by tossing his horn and demurely prancing to the music.

2. In 1869, the prosecution accused the youthful rebels of usurping the Cuban government.

3. Miss Hughes was no beauty; her value lay in her humor and an unusual knack of charming her pupils.

4. The stranger assured me the jewel was unique – the only puce ruby in Greater Dubuque.

5. The computer confused the scientists by its refusal to decide the issue with any and all of the usual answers.

6. I remained mute on the subject of Lester's new suit, which was a polluted green with flecks of liverish brown.

7. He got his education in the streets of Chicago, developing an astuteness he could never have learned in any university.

8. Eunice felt a thrill of curiosity as she and Jake sailed their craft, *Cupid's Arrow,* into the heart of the Bermuda Triangle.

9. The boy hid behind a huge statue of Zeus, enduring loneliness and boredom while waiting for the museum to close.

10. The duke halted the silly feud between the disputing clans and proclaimed the month of June a local holiday.

11. Every year Hubert made beautiful Yuletide candy shaped like musical instruments.

12. Hugo the Horrible used to sip bat juice and pick his teeth with barbecue skewers.

This exercise uses both $\overline{oo}$ and $\overline{u}$ sounds.

doves coo

owls ask "Who?"

termites chew

kittens mew

small boys glue

winners outdo

hairdressers shampoo

whales spew

Picasso drew

escapees think "Whew!"

cows moo

lumberjacks hew

lovers woo

(politicians too)

sleuths pursue

quitters are through

ghosts cry "Boo"

Gabriel blew

prompters cue

opiates subdue

blacksmiths shoe

skeptics say "Phoo"

nuts and bolts screw

operas debut

Lindberg flew

the beanstalk grew

friendships renew

payments are due

victims sue

critics review

witches brew

Bluebeard slew

losers rue

bills accrue

culprits stew

artists imbue

cynics eschew

flower girls strew

Garbo withdrew

Einstein knew

Winnie the Pooh

(as for me — I haven't a clue)

These sentences stress the vowel ô as in *off.*

1. The macaw was a raunchy sight due to its recent battle with our dog, Awful.

2. Paula's conversation was both frothy and gaudy and always sprinkled with great good humor.

3. The outlaw sure was a letdown: His jaw looked trembly and his horse had a cough.

4. I watched the moth with awe as it flitted high over the roaring waterfall.

5. We didn't realize how lonely Laurence was until he bought the ostrich.

6. Ora's eyes had a haunted look, almost as if she were recalling the night Brawley's ship was lost.

7. Kay paused in her song to wonder whether she had left Morton's socks at the laundromat.

8. Allen's warning message was scrawled in burnt cork on a wall near the crumbling altar.

9. The yellow shawl had fallen onto the floor of the hallway, and there in the sunlight it shone like a pool of gold.

10. The tawny-eyed girl slowly ate walnuts beneath the awning by a warm, green sea.

11. As I listened to his maudlin tale, I thought I ought to stifle my yawns, which threatened to become audible.

12. In Maudie's dream she was waltzing with a fawn that became a walrus on a broad expanse of whirling purple water.

These sentences stress the diphthong ī as in *ice*.

1. Ira's kite had a design of purple irises on an azure sky, and he certainly prized it.

2. To the scientist's surprise, the vine actually recognized him, raised a tendril, and tapped his right thumb.

3. The tide around the island was alive with dolphins, gliding side by side and chattering in the shiny sea.

4. Eli felt spry at 90 and still loved hiking up those icy crags roaring like a delighted mountain lion.

5. As the sacred ibis rose over the Nile, its wings a blur of white, I tried to describe it to my blind friend.

6. Eileen admired the mighty steed, a striped unicorn named Lionel, who wore a saddle of carved leather and ivory.

7. I am not wildly musical, though in kindergarten I once played the triangle and sometimes on Fridays I hum.

8. The nomads invited Heather into their tribe, calling her "Pride-of-the-Sun's-Eye."

9. As my glider took me soaring high above the pines, I realized this was my kind of paradise.

10. Yvonne cried, "I'm not a witch or a psychic!" — whereupon our long-silent clock chimed 85 times.

11. When Ida swiped my hair dryer, I was not polite and threatened to bite her canary's thigh.

12. Malcolm had hoped a constant diet of pies would blight his appetite for sweets, but every night he dreamed he was diving into pools of icing.

These sentences stress the diphthong *ou* as in *out*.

1. The Dowling family was astounded by their humble, profound giraffe.

2. Powell fooled around on the trumpet until he found his own unique sounds, which eventually earned him world renown.

3. The shrewd hound, jowls quivering and nose to the ground, soon located the convicts' treasure.

4. Sir Howard's house was surrounded by a moat with crimson flowers floating on it.

5. When the hour sounded, the crown toppled, and the tyrant's power was lost forever.

6. The old clown delighted the crowd with outrageous ways of falling down.

7. Janet's gown floated around her like a soft brown cloud.

8. The cheers for Robert Howell became so loud, he had to take a bow from the prow of the ship.

9. The countess was shrouded in a tower, drowsing and dreaming of the upcoming joust.

10. Poor Zu-Zu's dowry consisted of boundless good will from her parents, some cowry shells, and a pet mouse.

11. In a scene where she renounced her lover, the actress's bustle came loose and it bounced around until the audience howled.

12. Vowing revenge, the wizard mounted his horse and scoured the countryside for the enchanted owl.

These sentences stress the diphthong $\bar{o}$ as in *old*.

1. The ghost was doughy white and glowing softly as it floated across the drawing room and through the oaken door.

2. Joan held up her bandaged toe, saying she'd fallen into a shoal while hunting a clever blowfish on the Kona coast.

3. Miss Opal was thrilled when the zoning board voted to let her open a wax museum by the bowling alley.

4. We all felt a jolt when old Fuzzy Doakes left 40 cents to his wife and two million in gold to his goat, Patricia.

5. It was slow going through the snow, but they planned to reach the army post before another storm broke and wiped out the trail.

6. Nicole drew her cloak about her, thinking she heard Joseph roaming about somewhere below and wondered whether to make her presence known.

7. Grover shifted the heavy portfolio, hoping Mrs. Corey would notice him and ask to see his portraits of rodeo clowns.

8. The jovial crowd carried the heroic fireman around on their shoulders and later toasted him down at the local pub.

9. The only song I ever wrote was called "The Ballad of Goldy and Her Fat Old Moldy Toad."

10. "Please grow," I implored the reluctant orchid, a plant that specialized in moping and pouting.

11. Jonesy had been at the bottom of the totem pole for so long, he wondered how to cope with this startling success.

12. When Dorothy told stories of woeful events, she made them over to sound funny and we'd all roar; there were moments, too, when she forgot her loneliness and laughed with us.

These sentences stress the diphthong $\bar{a}$ as in *age*.

1. Our raven, Sadie, loved the penny arcade and even wanted to go there on rainy Sundays

2. Daisy McFay was frail, chaste, blameless, and a royal pain.

3. The first mate proudly unveiled his latest tattoo of Hudson Bay, which covered one shin and a kneecap.

4. James's amazing escapades during the race regaled the spectators, several of whom fainted.

5. The fireworks display at the Jade Pavilion brought acclaim and applause from the Chinese potentate.

6. The secret agent's holiday was endangered by bad breaks and a beautiful babe called Flame O'Shay.

7. The aliens came from a place they called "Roopa" near the constellation of Orion.

8. The actor in the play portrayed the old sage with a doddering grace until all Paris sang his praises.

9. Fabian the Arabian was a steed owned by the famous Geranium sisters who raced him at Churchill Downs.

10. Bob's painting showed an aging matriarch seated in the midst of her strange and tainted family.

11. In vain the shipwrecked sailors waited for the gale to abate, not knowing they huddled in the mouth of a live volcano.

12. The ruined cottage looked like a perfect haven to the escaping ape named Fenaday.

Selection

The last great Iji Island snail,
Eighty feet from head to tail,
Moved in stately, silent grace
Along its ancient, shaded trail.

These sentences stress the diphthong *oi* as in *boy*.

1. Doyle's clever plan foiled the villain, an oily fellow who enjoyed rat poison for breakfast.
2. The oyster sat in his bed, moistening and toying with the pearl he had just finished.
3. Roy's foibles finally reached the ears of his Aunt Joyce, who adroitly snipped him out of her will.
4. To Kermit's joy, the magic show was not spoiled by the threatening storm.
5. The noise of the amplified oboe inspired Mrs. Foy to raise her voice in song.
6. His hopes destroyed, the young boy nevertheless appeared poised before the jeering, boisterous crowd.
7. Elsa toiled over the embroidery for days, coiling a hidden message among the threads.
8. Boyd loitered by the guard's door, enjoying his chance to act as a decoy.
9. Helen of Troy was a royal wench who caused a good bit of annoyance when she was swiped by Paris, the boy wonder.
10. In 1890 Aunt Tessa made the difficult choice to leave her cloistered life as a doily maker and join Uncle Verne on his wild ranch near the Boise River.
11. After Pappy Boyle made a fortune in oysters, he purloined the rights to some hidden oil fields in Borneo.
12. She coyly grew her soybeans in window boxes all over Detroit.

SECTION B—SENTENCE QUOTATIONS

1. Happiness is a thing to be practiced, like the violin.
   Sir John Lubbock

2. Awake, arise, and stop not until the goal is reached.
   Upanishads

3. When one has much to put into them, a day has a hundred pockets.
   Nietzsche

4. The most completely lost of all days is the one on which we have not laughed.
   Chamfort

5. Merriment is a philosophy not well understood.
   Lord Byron

6. Man's joy or sorrow depends as much upon his disposition as upon his fate.
   La Rochefoucauld

7. As long as there are postmen, life will have zest.
   William James

8. I'm an optimist. It does not seem too much use being anything else.
   Winston Churchill

9. Society is frivolous, and shreds its days into scraps...
   Emerson

10. Even if I knew certainly the world would end tomorrow, I would plant an apple tree today.
    Martin Luther

11. To forgive a fault in another is more sublime than to be faultless one's self.
    George Sand

12. We must always change, renew, rejuvenate ourselves: Otherwise we harden.

Goethe

13. Every saint has a past and every sinner a future.

Kirpal Singh

14. He who knows his incapacity, knows something.

Marguerite De Valois

15. Unless you know yourself, the veil of delusion will not lift.

Nanak

16. It is only the jeweller's eye that at a glance can tell the ruby.

Bahi Nand Lal

17. Music is love in search of a word.

Sidney Lanier

18. The happiest person is the one who thinks the most interesting thoughts.

Timothy Dwight

19. The pleasures of thought are remedies for the wounds of the heart.

Mme. De Stael

20. Happy is the man who has broken the chains which hurt the mind, and has given up worrying once and for all.

Ovid

21. He deserves paradise who makes his companions laugh.

The Koran

22. Society would be a charming thing if we were only interested in one another.

Chamfort

23. Shun idleness: It is the rust that attaches itself to the most brilliant metals.

Voltaire

24. We shall all be perfectly virtuous when there is no longer any flesh on our bones.

Marguerite De Valois

25. To please, one must make up his mind to be taught many things which he already knows, by people who do not know them.

Chamfort

26. I do with my friends as I do with my books. I would have them where I can find them, but I seldom use them.

Emerson

27. The ornament of the house is the friends who frequent it.

Emerson

28. Can anybody remember when times were not hard and money not scarce?

Emerson

29. The beauty seen is partly in him who sees it.

Christian Bovee

30. Our deeds determine us as much as we determine our deeds.

George Eliot

31. Why are there trees I never walk under but large and melodious thoughts descend upon me?

Walt Whitman

32. Won't you come into my garden? I would like my roses to see you.

Richard Sheridan

33. Nothing great was ever achieved without enthusiasm.

Emerson

34. Truth is above all, but true living is still above truth.

Kirpal Singh

35. Whatever a man's age, he can reduce it several years by putting a bright-colored flower in his buttonhole.
Mark Twain

36. God that gives the wound may give the remedy. This is one day, but tomorrow is another...
Cervantes

37. Spirituality cannot be taught, it must be caught like an infection which is passed on to others who are receptive.
Kirpal Singh

38. True love is like a ghost: Everyone talks of it, but few have met it face to face.
La Rochefoucauld

39. A million speak of love, yet how few know, true love is not to lose remembrance even for an instant.
Kabir

40. Love bears all things, believes all things, hopes all things, endures all things, love never ends.
I. Corinthians

41. He that can have patience can have what he will.
Benjamin Franklin

42. All good fortune accrues to us when we have grown indifferent to it.
Proust

43. Conceal our passions as we may under the long cloaks of piety and honor, still will the cloven hoof peep out.
La Rochefoucauld

44. Contentment is better than riches, and a mind at peace with itself is worth more than the applause of assemblies.
Radhakrishnan

45. Our chief want in life is somebody who shall make us do what we can.

   Emerson

46. We have lived not in proportion to the number of years we have spent on the earth, but in proportion as we have enjoyed.

   Thoreau

47. To believe in a thing or fact without troubling to investigate it, does not in any way do credit to an intelligent man.

   Kirpal Singh

48. The existence of great souls is not suspected. They hide away: All that is seen is a little originality. There are more great souls than one would think.

   Stendhal

49. Take care, be careful, night and day look sharp...we do not stumble on mountains, but on clods, and fall.

   Chinese proverb

50. Life's but a walking shadow, a poor player that struts and frets his hour upon the stage and then is heard no more.

   Shakespeare

51. Give what you have. To someone, it may be better than you dare think.

   Longfellow

52. Walk on a rainbow trail: Walk on a trail of song, and all about you will be beauty. There is a way out of every dark mist, over a rainbow trail.

   Navajo song

53. The one remains, the many change and pass, life like a dome of many-colored glass, stains the white radiance of eternity.

Shelley

54. It is not fitting that I tell thee more, for the stream's bed cannot hold the sea.

Maulana Rumi

55. How does the sea become the king of all rivers and streams? Because it lies lower than them.

Lao Tse

56. Flowers are the moment's representations of things that are in themselves eternal.

Sri Aurobindo

57. He who would be humble regards himself as a student. He learns many new things, but what is more difficult, he unlearns many things he has learned.

Kirpal Singh

58. Let us treat men and women well: Treat them as if they were real: Perhaps they are.

Emerson

59. There is no odor so bad as that which arises from goodness tainted.

Thoreau

60. God implants guilt in a man, when he wishes to destroy a house utterly.

Aeschylus

61. If a man can be properly said to love something, it is the whole he loves and not merely parts of it.

Plato

62. It is good to tame the mind, which is difficult to hold in and flighty, rushing wherever it lists; a tamed mind brings happiness.

Buddha

63. The truth is that if you want a well governed state, you must find for your future rulers some career they like better than government. . .

Plato

64. Let my life be simple and straight like a flute of reed for thee to fill with music.

Tagore

65. The sooner you make your first five thousand mistakes, the sooner you will be able to correct them.

Nicolaides

66. To resist with success the frigidity of old age, one must combine the body, the mind, and the heart: To keep these in parallel vigor, one must exercise, study and love.

Bonstetten

67. The earth is not a mere fragment of dead history, stratum upon stratum like the leaves of a book, to be studied by geologists and antiquaries chiefly, but living poetry like the leaves of a tree, which precede flowers and fruit.

Thoreau

68. The human understanding is like a false mirror which receiving rays, irregularly distorts and discolors the nature of things by mingling its own nature with it.

Francis Bacon

69. The web of life is of a mingled yarn, good and ill together: Our virtues would be proud if our faults whipped them not: And our crimes would despair if they were not cherished by our virtues.

Shakespeare

70. But words are things, and a
        small drop of ink
    Falling, like dew, upon a
        thought produces
    That which makes thousands
        perhaps millions, think.
                                    Lord Byron

71. The moving finger writes: and, having writ,
    moves on; nor all thy piety nor wit
    shall lure it back to cancel half a line,
    nor all thy tears wash out a word of it.
                                    Omar Khayyam

72. How very commonly we hear it remarked that such
    and such thoughts are beyond the compass of words.
    I do not believe that any thought, properly so called,
    is out of the reach of language. For my own part, I have
    never had a thought which I could not set down in
    words, with ever more distinctness than that which I
    conceived it.
                                    Edgar Allan Poe

73. Morning air! If men will not drink of this at the foun-
    tainhead of the day, then we must bottle up some and
    sell it in the shops, for the benefit of those who have
    lost their ticket to morning time in this world.
                                    Henry David Thoreau

74. Your smile will inspire another to smile. Your strength
    will impel another to be strong. A noble soul always
    draws forth the noble quality in others.
                                    Kirpal Singh

Problems That May Arise

PURPOSE

Throughout the course of vocal rehabilitation you may observe that certain aspects of your treatment are more difficult than others. Many a patient has asked, "Why are words like *calm* and *olive* more difficult to practice than *meat* and *equal*?" Or: "Why do I sound so nasal since I have changed my pitch?" In answer to the first question, the difficulty lies in the stressed vowel within the word. The ä sound in *calm* and *olive* is produced at the back part of the mouth, while the ē sound of *meat* and *equal* is produced at the front part of the mouth. It is easier to maintain an optimal pitch level using the high front vowel sounds than it is the low back vowel sounds. In answer to the second question, the problem is one of balancing resonance. Often when the pitch is raised, too much nasality occurs and practice is necessary to obtain the desired vocal quality.

Your clinician also may hear certain problems that you do not detect. For example, the clinician might hear a grating sound or harshness that is produced only at the ends of sentences. This is caused by excessive tension at the vocal cord level. Monotony of delivery is also a common complaint, and in this instance vocal variety is lacking. Another problem is one of focus. Although pitch and tone focus are interrelated, there are times when the pitch is well established but the tone focus is still in the back of the throat, creating harshness or a lack of resonance. In these cases, the tone focus needs to be brought as far forward as possible into the mask of the face.

Another vocal problem that calls attention to a misused or abused voice is the glottal attack on words starting with a vowel. Easy initiation of sound is necessary to facilitate a pleasant-sounding voice and to secure vocal health.

Many questions are asked pertaining to volume, such as, "Why do I drop my pitch when speaking quietly?" There is a common tendency for people to use a low pitch during quiet, intimate conversation. This is unnecessary. When a person is speaking quietly, the desired voice is one in which the optimal or natural pitch is maintained, but the volume is lowered. Projection is the key here as it is when a louder voice is required. Professions such as acting or teaching place certain demands on the use of the voice, and a well-used voice can be heard in all kinds of situations. The development of these skills takes practice.

Everyone is different, which doesn't necessarily mean that each person will have one or more of these problems, but if a problem does arise similar to the ones mentioned, these vocal exercises often help to resolve it. Naturally, if you have no difficulty in these areas, this section can be omitted.

SECTION A—PROBLEM SOUNDS

GOAL To produce easily and clearly words that feature specific problem sounds.

PROCEDURE

1. Practice the following lists of words emphasizing the various stressed vowel sounds within the word. Continue to use your practice pitch.

2. Keep the tone focus as far forward as possible. Remember the mental picture of your imaginary target.

3. Follow through with the sentences that utilize the same sound.

The vowel ă as in *add* is the sound to be stressed in the following words.

Middle	Beginning
lamp	at
dance	an
spank	asp
band	ant
brash	ash
mask	ask
chance	anchovy
cackle	anagram
prattle	angle
cactus	apple
fatten	after
grapple	anguish
ramble	ample
sanction	actor
baffle	anchor
manta ray	angry
sampan	asteroid
cattle	alchemy
taffeta	altitude
master	abracadabra

These sentences stress the vowel sound ă as in *add*.

1. The pampered hamster nibbled on brandied apples and coconuts from Honolulu.

2. Miss Blanche's taffeta gown made such a racket I had to strain to catch what the actors were saying.

3. The sampan rolled down the Yangtze River, steered by a crew of bandits wearing dragon masks.

4. The jasmine tree was aghast when the man announced it was nothing but sap and chlorophyll.

5. Bash Bennett's ray gun zapped open the hidden cabinet and revealed a cache of black pearls.

6. Madam Manton eyed the Andes peak as if it were just an anthill and said she'd reach the top crag on Saturday.

7. The jazz dancer leaped with great dash and a madly wicked grin.

8. Grandpa rambled on about that night in January 1928, when Mademoiselle Gigi taught him the fandango.

9. The alchemist muttered "Abracadabra!" and turned the brass candlesticks into gold.

10. Practical Anne married the richest land baron in Brazil and then spent several years mapping the Amazon River.

11. Astronaut Crandall sat on the shadowy planet with a nagging suspicion that he was not alone.

12. Allen practiced his magic act for many years before stocking up on some brand new rabbits and tackling Broadway.

The vowel ä as in *father* is the sound to be stressed in the following words.

Middle	Beginning
far	ox
palm	arm
heart	optimist
clop	otter
blob	option
calm	honest
fox	oblong
guard	archery
psalm	arduous
carved	optic
clock	artist
star	onyx
jolly	honor
cotton	octave
pocket	homage
garden	olive
possible	arctic
copper	octopus
bothered	armor
harmless	oddity

These sentences stress the vowel sound ä as in *father*.

1. Art's father was the calmest bronco buster in Otter Tail, Wyoming.

2. The dog trudged through the Arctic snow, wishing Mr. McCarty would shout something more heartening than "Mush!"

3. My iguana's name is Godzilla Garcia, and he is an optimist.

4. Grandfather believed a sharp wit and a wise heart were the best qualities possible in a bartender.

5. In 1612, the onyx box was carried on an arduous journey to the court of the great Aga Khan.

6. Martha was a copper-haired beauty who sang opera as she tended her ant farm.

7. The potter leaned down and presto! — he formed a teapot from the olive-colored clay.

8. The ox team pulled out a carful of damp and snarling travelers from the muddy stream.

9. Carl's ardor for chimes delighted his papa who hoped the boy would major in doorbell repair.

10. Barbara's G above high C shattered the crystal on Dr. Armstrong's charming old watch.

11. The octopus often thought back to those carefree days under the reef before she was captured by the aquanauts.

12. Oliver had a jolly time at the optometrist's ball; he led the conga line and then danced into the dawn doing his famous box step.

The vowel ŭ as in *up* is the sound to be stressed in the following words.

Middle	Beginning
bum	us
slush	up
gloves	ulcer
flood	under
love	other
crumb	onion
bust	uncle
frump	upper
drum	ultimate
cult	ugly
fudge	umpire
stunned	oven
fussy	uppity
mummy	unction
vulnerable	undercover
culture	utmost
pungent	utterly
gullible	usher
vulgar	ultra
lucky	undulate

These sentences stress the vowel sound ŭ as in up.

1. Aunty Belle insisted on hugging Rusty and calling him "Sweet Lovey-Dovey" whenever she visited us in Council Bluffs.

2. The culprit hid the freshly stolen pumpkin under his dusty cloak and then asked the way to Bumblebee Creek.

3. The ugliest pup I ever saw was named Sludge, but he was no dummy, and his heart was as big as an oven.

4. Professor Taylor made a wonderful lunchtime punch of cucumbers and white wine.

5. The truck lumbered toward the Puffy Pillow Factory with a cargo of five hundred indignant ducks.

6. Mr. Lundy lost his temper whenever he thought of the public's unjust treatment of buzzards.

7. The grubby youngster looked up, cupping his hands to receive a few drops from the thunderstorm.

8. Hulda believed occult powers would change her from a gullible frump into a stunning undercover agent.

9. Scuttlebutt had it that our chum Duffy had taken the plunge with a plump little number from Buffalo.

10. I thought if Duncan said "a rum go" one more time, I would crush the tea rose in his buttonhole.

11. In the tiny club, Marlene thumped away at her drums, unaware that she was creating quite a hubbub.

12. Bud wrote that he was adjusting to the rough instructions from his superiors and that he no longer felt like a wrung-out dunce.

SECTION B—NASALITY

GOAL   To eliminate any nasality that may have developed as a result of the changeover into the correct pitch and tone focus.

PROCEDURE

1. The words on the following page contain vowels and/or diphthongs that some people have a tendency to nasalize.

2. As you repeat the words pay close attention to the stressed vowel and/or diphthong.

3. Be sure the soft palate is raised (your clinician can show you) as you blend from a consonant into the vowel. Also, use care when blending from a vowel into a nasal sound (m, n, ng).

4. Follow through with the sentences. The method of practice is noted on each page of the sentence drill.

Word drill to eliminate nasality

The columns of words may be read downward, thus segregating the "no nasals" from the "nasals," or across by alternating them.

No nasal	Nasal	No nasal	Nasal
rag	band	couch	crown
cap	clam	sprout	round
dally	antler	foul	pounce
ladder	stranded	loud	township
raffle	channel	tower	bounty
palace	scramble	power	scoundrel

No nasal	Nasal
guide	wine
pride	chime
fight	rhyme
write	mind
plight	grind
ride	climb

Sentences to eliminate nasality

The following sentences have no nasal sounds in them. An interesting way to practice is to first read them while gently holding your nose. No pressure should be felt. If there is pressure, make efforts to raise the soft palate higher on the vowels and diphthongs. Next, read the sentences naturally, without the pressure on the nose. Tape-record both ways if possible. The quality of the voice should sound the same regardless of whether the nose is held or not.

1. The stray cat was black with eyes of electric blue.

2. Dale thought the cat was a gorgeous beast: It had a bold swagger to its walk.

3. He called the creature Fearless Fosdick (Foz for short). All that August they both explored the wild hillside forests where they scaled oak trees or cliff tops with the speed of cheetahs.

4. The two were always together: Foz slept atop Dale's pillow, face to face with the child.

5. Dale's sister said, "That cat will get restless, you'll see. He'll disappear. After all, he's just a stray." She was a rather callous sort.

6. But Foz stayed. He loved to swagger through the breezy gusts of October. His greatest hour, however, was the happy vigil by Dale's doorway as they greeted trick-or-treaters who thought Foz was a perfect All Hallow's Eve cat.

A good vocal quality should be balanced among the three resonating cavities — the nose, the mouth, and throat. Some nasal resonance is needed, however, and should not be confused with nasality, which is caused by too much nasal resonance. Read the following sentences remembering to keep the tone focus as far forward in the mask of the face as possible.

1. Whenever Dinah Dowling pounded a nail, her left thumb expected the worst.

2. Little Dinah was accident prone; while screwing taps on her tap shoes, she had managed to attach her left index finger instead.

3. Dinah's howl was heard down the entire block. It took a pediatrician and a shoe repair man 30 minutes to loosen Dinah from the tap shoe.

4. One day when her cousin, Melanie Ann Dratt, arrived to play, Dinah suggested they climb a giant fir tree to look for eagles' nests. Just as they reached the top, a 60-mile-an-hour wind came up, bending the tree far out over Lake Booney.

5. The girls clung to the top branches, which whapped furiously back and forth in an aerial ballet of tree tops, legs, arms, bloomers, and screams.

6. Finally Mr. and Mrs. Dowling missed the girls and, without wasting a moment, phoned the fire department and their old friend, Chief Lambert, whom they had met the night Dinah got her foot caught in the toilet.

7. Chief Lambert said, "Okay, where's the worst place Dinah could be during a high wind?" Together both parents looked toward the giant fir tree.

8. When the wind died down, rescue operations began, but it was another hour before both girls were safely on the ground again; all the while Melanie Ann had been debating whether she wanted to continue being Dinah's cousin.

9. Late that afternoon the two children were enjoying some lime sherbet, while everyone else breathed a huge sigh of relief. In fact, they were all sighing so hard, nobody but Melanie Ann heard Dinah whisper, "Hey, I know what let's do now!" And with that, every drop of color drained out of poor Melanie's face.

SECTION C—HARSHNESS

The r and l sounds have been known to create harshness in the voice if they occur at the ends of words or when the tone focus falls too far back in the throat.

GOAL To eliminate any excessive tension at the vocal fold level that might cause a harsh sound to be heard at the ends of words and sentences.

PROCEDURE

1. When practicing either the r or the l sound, make efforts to utter the word in a sliding scale. For example:

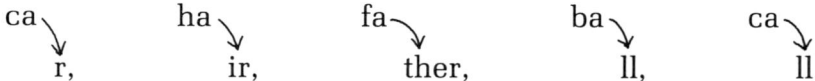

As the final sound or syllable is uttered, the pitch drops, but the tone focus must be kept forward. Again, your imaginary target may help you to accomplish this. The words should be clear, regardless of the drop in pitch.

2. Follow through with the sentences that emphasize /r/ and /l/ at the ends of words.

R is the sound to be stressed in the following words as you slide down the scale vocally.

End	Middle
pear	fierce
veer	rural
tear	north
dear	dwarf
tore	mirth
spar	born
care	cheered
moor	forest
burr	carriage
rare	charmer
score	mournful
jeer	surely
lair	arid
spear	married
lore	porridge
jar	market
tour	caring
aware	parent
career	arrow
mirror	hurry

These sentences stress the sound of r.

1. Rennie researched storms: Her specialty was hurricanes, but she also loved gentle summer showers.

2. The rocket raced toward the far-off star with a crew determined to reach the speed of light.

3. Astride her horse, cantering through Central Park, Robin adored those brilliant April mornings.

4. The dancer's earrings sparkled in the light of her campfire, as she whirled to the strains of the Spanish guitar.

5. The truck reached Glacier Park as the sun burst into view over the rim of Razor Mountain.

6. The courtiers stared as the juggler scattered emeralds over the marble floor.

7. The gardener coaxed the fern to uncurl itself, rewarding it with a mulch of orchid sprouts.

8. Heather charmed her father as she described her adventures in Morocco with the nomad tribe.

9. Roger wondered why the fishermen ran in terror, for he considered himself a very friendly sea serpent.

10. The rider's eyes explored the gray and gold Sahara, trying to make out the hidden trails of caravans.

11. Greg pursued the apparition through the forest until he stumbled upon a barn with its door ajar.

12. The archer raised his bow and arrow, and like a mythical figure he stood ready, his shadow reflected in the water.

L is the sound to be stressed in the following words as you slide down the scale vocally.

End	Middle
sail	gulp
fool	cold
smile	jilt
kneel	scald
yell	shelve
doll	realm
male	golf
duel	silk
trill	solve
drool	film
coil	help
snail	tilt
troll	scalp
eel	palace
gargle	calling
novel	gallant
saddle	ballad
ladle	tailor
giggle	yellow
tattle	stalled

These sentences stress the sound of *l*.

1. Rudolph Valentino once lived in a fabulous palace called Falcon's Lair.

2. Her name was Velvet Lee O'Grady, this luscious, strange, elusive lady.

3. The elders told the space traveler that Vulcan is a planet located on the far side of the sun.

4. Gulliver's adventures in Lilliput turned Lady Edith's lonely evenings into special events, both sparkling and delightful.

5. Dell's poor, tangled memories began to unravel with galling slowness, until he finally recalled the man who betrayed him.

6. Ham and Shem admired their dad's talent for building arks and collecting livestock.

7. In the novel, the doll sprang to life, doing back flips and cartwheels the whole night long.

8. Why are platypuses difficult to love? — animal experts admit this is a stickler.

9. The mystery revolved around a latchkey, some yellowed lace, and a Balinese bowl.

10. Noel was quickly becoming a legend on his unicycle, as he peddled along the top of the castle wall.

11. Lillian wished her weird Uncle Cal would not tickle her, yell "You old bag!" and run off with a giggle.

12. The fortune that Estelle sought was rumored to be a hill of solid gold deep in the jungle of Brazil.

SECTION D—PITCH DISCRIMINATION

GOAL To develop confident pitch discrimination and to increase vocal variety.

PROCEDURE

1. Read each sentence three times using appropriate volume. The first time read the sentence on the pitch level just *above* your natural pitch. The second time read the sentence on your natural pitch level, and the third time read the sentence on the pitch just *below* your natural level. For example:

   This exercise is fine. (one note above)
   This exercise is fine. (natural pitch)
   This exercise is fine. (one note below)

   Or you may start on your *natural* pitch and then read the sentence one note *above* your natural pitch, come back to your *natural* pitch, and finally to one note *below*.

2. Each sentence should be read at a moderate rate and with as little vocal variety as possible within the sentence. This method is used to sharpen your pitch discrimination.

3. The tone focus must be kept forward at all times throughout this exercise.

4. For another variation read each sentence on a different pitch level. Start from your highest, most comfortable level and descend one note at a time until you have said the sentence at your lowest, most comfortable level. If you feel any strain, stop your practice. You may be going beyond your vocal range. Only four or five notes may be possible at this stage, but with practice you may develop a range of one octave or more. Vocal variety increases with practice, and this is one exercise that may be of value.

These sentences stress pitch discrimination.

1. I wish spring would hurry.
2. The volcano spewed forth its flames.
3. This year I'm sailing to Greece.
4. My monkey plays the harp.
5. Not all elves are shoemakers.
6. October is the month for opals.
7. My sister swam the English channel.
8. Breezes force the trees to gossip.
9. Penguins seldom brush their teeth.
10. Vampires look forward to sunset.
11. I'd like to ride on a comet.
12. Did you hear what that dolphin said?
13. The nightingale's song drifted slowly away.
14. The narrow, deep gorges filled me with awe.
15. A centaur is a most remarkable creature.
16. The giant's smile melted my fear.
17. The old fallen log housed a family of trolls.
18. Listen to the silence and tell me what you hear.
19. The story the raven told was hard to believe.
20. Riding in a hansom takes one back in time.
21. The leprechauns were caught dancing in the moonlight.
22. When an eagle comes all the sparrows fly away.

SECTION E—TONE FOCUS

GOAL   To develop the correct tone focus in the mask of the face.

PROCEDURE

1. Exercise I, the humming exercise, helps you to experience mask-of-the-face tone focus. As you practice it, your attention should be on the vibrations created in the lips and teeth by vigorous humming.

2. In reversing the exercise, you will find that the sensation of the vowel is not as strong as the hum. Nevertheless, practice placing the vowel as far forward in the mask of the face as possible. This exercise will help you to tune in to the subtleties of focus in spontaneous speech.

3. To complete the exercise, follow through with the word list and the sentences.

4. Exercises II, III, and IV also help in alerting you to the feeling of a correct tone focus. Producing the sound of the consonant *w* in a rhythmic way activates the lips, thereby calling attention to a forward sensation. Not only should "wah," "way," "wee," etc., be initiated easily, but the lips should be free of tension as well.

5. The word list and sentences incorporate two sounds, *w* and *hw*. Both these sounds are produced in the same way, although *w* is voiced and *hw* is unvoiced. But as far as the exercise is concerned, both are mutually helpful.

6. As in Exercise I, follow through with the words and sentences.

Humming exercise

EXERCISE I   Hum on the *m* sound until you feel your lips vibrating. Continue until it takes up about half your breath supply, and then go gently into the following vowel sounds. Repeat each one three times.

M-m-m	OO	M-m-m	$\overline{\text{I}}$
M-m-m	OH	M-m-m	$\overline{\text{A}}$
M-m-m	AH	M-m-m	$\overline{\text{E}}$

It is important to blend the humming sound into the following vowel as if you were speaking a word. For example, mmmooo, not mmm (pause) oo. The same holds true for the reversal of Exercise I.

Reverse Exercise I, chanting the vowel first on your natural pitch level and ending with a prolonged hum. Again, remember that the inner sensation of the vowel is not as strong as the hum. Repeat each one three times.

OO	M-m-m	$\overline{\text{I}}$	M-m-m
OH	M-m-m	$\overline{\text{A}}$	M-m-m
AH	M-m-m	$\overline{\text{E}}$	M-m-m

Words and sentences stressing the *m* sound

Hum on the beginning *m* sound and then vocally move gently into the remainder of the word. For example, m-m...eal.

meal	monster	motor
mean	mongrel	molar
measles	moon	maid
meager	moor	mail
mince	moose	maize
mint	moody	mayhem
minister	mute	major
mimic	mutual	mild
meld	mutism	mime
meadow	mutiny	mind
meditate	maul	migrate
medley	mourn	minus
mad	moss	mound
map	maudlin	mouth
magnet	mope	mouse
manage	mole	mountain
mop	moan	moist
mob	moment	moisture

Hum only on the beginning *m* sound in the first word of each sentence. Then proceed in speaking the rest of the sentence naturally.

1. My aunt's macadamia nut pie was famous on the island of Maui.

2. Much to my surprise no one cared for Merton's musical tribute to mermaids.

3. Madge amazed us with her imitations of Minnie Mouse and Marilyn Monroe.

4. Moneybags, our mynah, sang Mexican songs while I played the maracas.

5. Many of us thought that Myrna wasn't much prettier than her pet ostrich.

6. Marvin's grandfather was the greatest magician in Moose Lip, Alaska.

7. Mitzi McGee liked to make monkey faces behind the mayor's back.

8. Mark my word, any man who plays tag with sharks won't live to see Monday.

9. Mr. Moto, the famous detective, matched wits with many a criminal mastermind.

10. "Memorizing the Gettysburg Address," sighed Miss Mae, "is almost as hard as trying to remember it."

11. Midnight Madness was the fastest mare I ever rode into the winner's circle.

12. "Maybe you can go out tomorrow night, Son," said the werewolf's mother, "when the moon isn't so full."

Poem

My bandages may be loose and crummy,
But I'm still Mildred's favorite mummy.

Exercises stressing the *w* sound

EXERCISE II   At your practice pitch, repeat the following exercise rapidly but lightly eight to ten times.

wah   way   wee   wi   woh   woo

EXERCISE III   Gently and easily slide down the scale with each nonsense syllable, keeping the tone focus forward in the mask of the face.

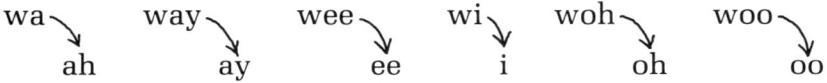

Be careful as you go into the lower pitch range that the tone focus doesn't slip into the back of the throat. Regardless of pitch, the tone focus must always be in the mask of the face.

EXERCISE IV   Using *wah way wee wi woh woo*, start at your highest, most comfortable pitch level, and come down the scale to your lowest, most comfortable pitch level, keeping the tone focus as far forward as possible. The speaking voice should be used and not the singing voice.

wah   way   wee   wi   woh   woo
    wah   way   wee   wi   woh   woo
        wah   way   wee   wi   woh   woo
            wah   way   wee   wi   woh   woo, etc.

Note: This exercise can also be practiced substituting the sound of /m/ for /w/.

Word pairs stressing *w* and *hw*

Overarticulate as you read each pair of words and be aware of the difference between the voiced *w* and the voiceless *hw*.

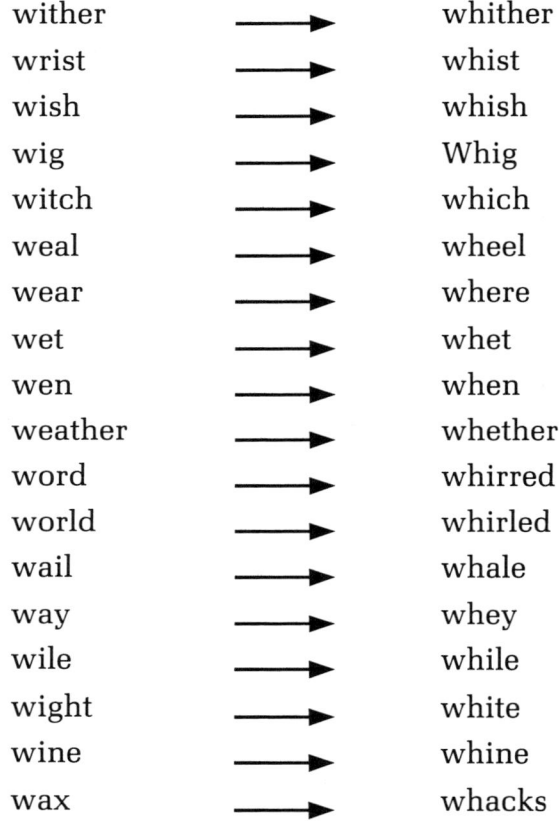

wither	⟶	whither
wrist	⟶	whist
wish	⟶	whish
wig	⟶	Whig
witch	⟶	which
weal	⟶	wheel
wear	⟶	where
wet	⟶	whet
wen	⟶	when
weather	⟶	whether
word	⟶	whirred
world	⟶	whirled
wail	⟶	whale
way	⟶	whey
wile	⟶	while
wight	⟶	white
wine	⟶	whine
wax	⟶	whacks

Sentences stressing *w* and *hw* contrast

As you read the following sentences, you will notice a strong movement of your lips produced by the repetition of the *w* and *hw* sounds. The exercise is meant to keep your attention in the front of your mouth rather than at the back of your throat.

w

1. All Waldo wanted was to win something, anything, just once.
2. On her wilder rides, Wanda the witch caught her skirts on our weather vane.
3. "If you wind your clocks too tightly," William warned, "time will certainly stop."
4. After Olive ran off with the window washer, Wendell put away his dancing shoes.

hw

1. Whitcomb loved to film whales from a whirlybird.
2. "Who, what, when, where, and why" is the journalist's motto.
3. Whitey failed to whet my appetite with his whipped prune and clam dip.
4. Grandpa used to whittle tiny whimsical creatures while he told us stories about them.

w and *hw*

1. My first line was: "Whither will we go, dear Willard?"— whereupon I quit.
2. We used to see Wilcox down by the wharves pushing his wife in a wheelbarrow.
3. Oh, she was a whirlwind, all right, when she first worked at the wicker factory.
4. Old Willy whistled through his whiskers as he went to woo Miss Witherspoon.

SECTION F—GLOTTAL ATTACK

GOAL   To avoid glottal attacks on words that start with a vowel and to bring under control an easy initiation of sound.

PROCEDURE

1. As you practice the following exercises, be careful to initiate the voice in a smooth, relaxed manner. The voicing should feel as if it is effortless. This will prevent vocal fold abuse.

2. Take notice of how the glottal attack is eliminated as you move quickly through the h sound into the following vowel within the word.

Exercises to eliminate the glottal attack

EXERCISE I Say the following words gently. You will observe that all the words start with an *h* sound. This sound before a vowel helps to bring your vocal folds together without excessive tension.

he	hot	hood
heel	hock	hook
heat	hop	hoof
heap	hall	high
heed	halter	hide
hit	haunt	height
hinge	hawk	hike
hilt	hull	how
hip	hut	howl
help	hulk	hound
hence	hush	house
helm	whose	hole
hem	hoop	hope
hat	who	host
hack	hoot	hoyle
hand	whom	hoist

EXERCISE II   In the following pairs of words initiate the word starting with a vowel as smoothly as you do when pronouncing the word that starts with the *h* sound.

heat — eat	hair — air
heel — eel	hear — ear
hit — it	hall — all
his — is	halter — alter
hid — id	hush — usher
hill — ill	whose — ooze
helm — elm	hoops — oops
Hester — Esther	hive — I've
hat — at	hide — I'd
ham — am	high — eye
hand — and	hike — Ike
had — add	hire — ire
has — as	how — ow
hash — ash	howl — owl
heart — art	hold — old
harden — Arden	hone — own
harbor — arbor	hate — ate
harm — arm	hail — ail
hark — ark	hoyle — oil

EXERCISE III   Each sentence starts with the *h* sound to assist in the recall of relaxed phonation. This will also help you to carry over the skills of blending from one word into another starting with a vowel.

1. Harold adored telegrams.
2. Hop in, Miss Macintosh!
3. Hamlets are found in Denmark.
4. Helen always smirks in church.
5. How are your scuba lessons?
6. Hum it and I'll chime in.
7. Hardy is he who eats nails.
8. Heaven is her cat's name.
9. Hannah's anklet was gorgeous.
10. Have another macaroon.
11. Hairdos are a source of grief.
12. Herbert's ox ate my tamale.
13. Holly is a Christmas name.
14. Humphrey either loves you or he doesn't.
15. Her ivy is awfully happy.
16. Hold onto your socks, Tilly!
17. Hands across the sea get wet.
18. He's under the car just now.
19. Who asked for marzipan?
20. Hiram and Bess are eels.

EXERCISE IV   These sentences offer an opportunity to practice blending naturally into words that start with a vowel. When the first word in the sentence starts with a vowel, speak the word easily to avoid the glottal attack.

1. Arlene always enjoyed surprises involving okra.

2. If you ever get out to Rangoon, give us a call.

3. Each August the asters on her hat would bloom.

4. Ed mailed dozens of pet anchovies to lonely shut-ins.

5. An angry armadillo is not my idea of excitement.

6. Odd how rare encouragement is, and it's so inexpensive, too!

7. In April and October I'm most affected by the changing light.

8. Every summer Effie entered the annual log-rolling contest.

9. Oakley was usually all set to show off his antique umbrellas.

10. Honestly, I marvel at how often Arvid has ignored defeat.

11. Apples are named everything from All-over-red to Sparkler crab to Pocomoke.

12. In his eightieth year, Uncle Al battled the treacherous white water of Arrow Gorge.

SECTION G—VOLUME

GOAL To gain control in the appropriate use of volume.

PROCEDURE

1. Be sure to use midsection breath support while executing these exercises and mentally connect the breath with the sound in the hard palate.

2. In Exercises I through V, no strain should be felt in the vocal fold area if the voice is supported by correct breathing and focused in the mask of the face. If you begin to feel any strain whatever, please stop practicing and consult your clinician.

3. The practice pitch should be maintained during the practice of the following exercises whether you are using full projection or speaking quietly.

Exercises for projection

EXERCISE I The value of this exercise is derived from the use of your practice pitch, correct tone focus, easy initiation of sound, and midsection breathing. When you feel confident that you are controlling the voice at the practice pitch, you may then use your optimal pitch to accomplish this exercise. The feeling of balanced resonance should be unmistakable. Do not push for volume, but allow it to grow naturally with your practice, and avoid using a low pitch or throat resonance.

        ho-ho 1
        ho-ho 2
        ho-ho 3 (continue through 10)

        ho-ho 1   ho 1
        ho-ho 2   ho 2
        ho-ho 3   ho 3 (continue through 10)

ho   1 (continue through 10)

In practicing this next step, which is more difficult, the h sound is dropped. Initiate the *oh* as smoothly as possible in order to avoid any harshness. It will help if the soft palate is raised as much as possible.

oh-oh 1 (through 10)
oh-oh 1   oh 1 (through 10)
oh 1   (through 10)

Follow this exercise with the words stressing the *oh* diphthong in Step Two and the sentences stressing the *oh* diphthong in Step Three.

EXERCISE II   Say each sentence twice. The first time use full projection and when you repeat the sentence, speak as softly as possible. Maintain your optimal pitch level throughout the exercise. You may use your optimal pitch level with the following exercise if you are absolutely sure of it. If not, continue using your practice pitch.

JANUARY WEARS WHITE.
January wears white.

FEBRUARY GLOWERS.
February glowers.

MARCH BRINGS PUDDLES.
March brings puddles.

APRIL SENDS FLOWERS.
April sends flowers.

MAY DRESSES UP.
May dresses up.

JUNE KICKS OFF HER SHOES.
June kicks off her shoes.

JULY GOES OUT A-TRAVELING.
July goes out a-traveling.

WHILE AUGUST TAKES A SNOOZE.
While August takes a snooze.

SEPTEMBER REAPS THE HARVEST.
September reaps the harvest.

OCTOBER PAINTS WITH GOLD.
October paints with gold.

NOVEMBER FEATURES TURKEYS.
November features turkeys.

DECEMBER LOVES THE COLD.
December loves the cold.

EXERCISE III   The first part of the sentence should be read as if you were speaking to a large audience. Then utter the second part of the sentence as softly as possible *without* dropping your pitch.

1. I DO CARTWHEELS
   in my spare time.

2. BY GUM, WHAT A PLUM!
   I'm glad we won.

3. THE CROCODILE SMILED
   then sneaked away.

4. THE SHUTTER WAS FLAPPING
   on one rusty hinge.

5. BRENT LIKES MICE
   better than me.

6. PANSY LOU SEES SPOTS
   when she crosses her eyes.

7. THE PIGEON SWOOPED DOWN
   and brought us the message.

8. POOR OLD McPEEP,
   he's asleep in the deep.

9. WE HEARD THE PARROT CALL
   across the marble hall.

10. PAMPAS GRASS IS SHARP
    with razor green leaves.

11. THE WIND MOANS LOW
    over Pirate's Bay.

12. ZORA WORE SCARLET
    to the Witches' Ball.

13. MYRNA CRACKED THE CODE
    in four minutes flat.

14. THE TIRED OLD ROBOT
    smiled his rusty smile.

15. I ONCE MET A MARTIAN
    with small green toes.

16. THE WILD RED POPPIES
    blew toward the south.

Paragraphs

EXERCISE IV   Read the following selections with your projected voice.

The Circus

Good evening and welcome, children of all ages. The Greatest Show on Earth will make this a night each of you will find unforgettable—a night filled with fantastic feats, performed for you with surpassing grace and courage by the most daring men and women in the world. Carlo the Magnificent will stop your breath with his lethal harem of Bengal tigers; The Flying Alonzos will soar and whirl fifty feet above the glittering sand; and Princess Fifi will dance across a tiny silver wire with her famous python, Sinbad. All this and more, much more — elephants, bears, horses from the Arabian deserts, clowns to delight you, acrobats and jugglers to amaze you; Bruno, a fire-eating strongman, and the Ming Brothers, twin magicians from the deepest recesses of the Orient. And so I say welcome, my friends, welcome one and all to the Greatest Show on Earth.

The Lottery

I just won the state lottery. Hear that? Four million dollars. I am rich, wealthy, moneyed, loaded, rolling in bucks, overflowing, profuse, and doing pretty well, thank you.

Here is a list of the things I will leave behind forever: holes in my underwear, "overdue" notices, baggy sofas, graffiti on my stove, drooping curtains, plastic orchids, sassy roaches, patched tires, my job painting curbs, my landlady, my 1966 Rambler, and Aunt Gert. She always said, "You're a dreamer and a schemer, but you'll never scrape up enough change to buy thumbtacks." So long, Aunt Gert. I'll send you a box of little sharp things to play with.

Now here's a list of what's in my future: a house in Jamaica, sky diving, entirely new teeth, pedicures, white velvet upholstery, balloon rides, tumbling lessons, breakfast serenades, rum baba in Paris, Mardi Gras in Venice, adventure on the Orient Express, my own carousel, cashmere pajamas, a portrait of myself in stained glass, pet baby giraffes, and a private entrance to my car.

Are you ready for me, world? Are you prepared? I sure hope so, because I'm not waiting around another second. Get set! He-e-e-re I come!

The Giant

What do you mean, I'm loud? All giants are loud. Whoever heard of a quiet giant? I'm loud and proud of it. Even my hair is loud. When I walk, the earth shudders and groans, birds fly around like crazy, animals stampede, bees and hornets run into each other, and sometimes even trees fall down. I can't help making a stir. That's what giants are for: to stir things up, get things moving, make a commotion. The world's so involved with little, no-account piffles, like where did the car keys go or how come the plumbing's backed up again — stuff like that.

Well, giants are here to interrupt, to make people look up instead of down all the time. We love to see change and something different happening. But, no matter how it seems, we're not careless. We don't just run around willy-nilly tearing things apart. No, as we're piling up new mountain ranges or digging out fresh beds for the ocean, we're thinking ahead to see what our remodeling's going to mean in the long run.

So, stop complaining about how loud or disruptive we are, because we're the shakers and the movers and the doers. We're the future right here in the present. We're giants!

EXERCISE V   The next selections may be read quietly, but the pitch should be at its optimal level or slightly above, the voice clear, and the speech audible as if someone were listening to you. Do not whisper.

When I'm Old

Someday when I'm old and no one cares where I go or what I do, I will live by this stream, instead of only visiting once in a while. I'll wake to its busy, bubbly sound and spend my days watching speckled trout and crayfish, blue dragonflies, and the stick-like insects called "skippers" skimming across the water's surface. Here I'll sit, warm and drowsy, quiet and content, and as the Indians say, "old and covered with my life." The roar of my battles will be behind me; victories and losses will all have drifted off. By then I believe I shall be ready for silence, that silence which I know lies both above and beneath my existence, and surrounds all the annoying, strident sounds in my life. I shall hear it clearly then, and put myself in the midst of it, drawing it around me like a soft, feathery cloak...

So here I'll be when I'm old, here by the stream, smiling and resting and finished with noise. Why don't you come see me then? Sit down, too, and we'll both watch the stream and be companions sharing the day, the dragonflies, and the silence.

The Desert

The desert quiets me. There's no clamor out here, no motors or roars or growls — even the wolves have gone north. The absence of birds also causes a quiet not found in other regions, and it's typical of the place that the most dreaded sound is a snake's rattle. Here, noise is a stranger.

When you're used to them, sounds can be a comfort — companions, in a way. But the desert is a place for those who don't need much reassurance. And part of adjusting to it is accepting its silence. Something else is necessary, too — catching on to its sense of humor — mirages, for instance. Out here the most ordinary thing, like a pond, is recreated into an illusion that's totally convincing. Visions of ponds have tempted me to keep walking far beyond any point that's safe. I've seen trees beside the water and horses, even tents. Luckily I've realized in time I'd better turn back. If I'd gone on, I'd have moved straight into an inferno.

There are mirages here for the ears, too. One day I thought I heard the distant ring of bells — sleigh bells, of all things. And music when the wind reaches a certain pitch. To break these fantasies I talk to myself and my dog, Sadie. A voice will bring back reality.

Being alone out here, I depend on certain things to stay in touch with what I know is solid. The sounds I make are deliberate, and I keep Sadie near me because her movements strengthen my sense of self. It's a comfort to hear her lie down or lap water.

The best moments come after the long, hot day when she and I entertain ourselves. Sometimes we harmonize on "Pop Goes the Weasel"; I sing alto while she howls soprano. Other nights, by the light of the kerosene lamp, I read to her, my voice making a path through the shadows. And there is a contentment we feel then, in just the two of us coping with the desert. Somehow we've made our own way in this solitary, defiant place. To us, it's beautiful and because of that, we belong to it.

Someday

Today is my fiftieth birthday and everyone tells me I have to stop waiting for Someday. My whole life long I've waited for Someday, trying to ignore the mundane, boring todays, thinking, Someday I'll lose weight and fix up my apartment and be able to afford a good car. Someday I'll start exercising. My skin will smooth out and my eyesight will improve because I'll be eating lots of carrots. I don't like carrots now, but I will Someday. I'll have a torso like a Spanish dancer's from all my exercising, and I won't be so bashful anymore. In fact, I'll have developed confidence; no, better than that, wit. People will burst out laughing at the things I say. If I meet a rich couple, they may ask me to cruise the Mediterranean with them on their yacht. For breakfast I'll sip champagne with a strawberry in it, and I'll swim off the coast of Sardinia. And as I traipse through the great casino at Monte Carlo, with everyone laughing at the outrageous comments I make, I'll suddenly look over to see two intense, sable-colored eyes staring right into mine. Though they'll be the eyes of a stranger, there will also be something familiar about them . . . "Isn't Fate strange?" I'll think, for the eyes will belong to a tall, pirate-faced man, leaning against a pillar. Only . . . only he's stopped leaning now, and he's begun to walk toward me with the confidence of someone used to gliding past patrol boats at midnight. . . . And I? Without hesitation I leave my companions who can't quite realize what's happening. But other people do, and they turn to stare. I don't care. Neither does he. We move toward each other, part of the same spell. . . .

Oh, no. No. That can't be the phone. What time is it? Six P.M. . . . Cousin Molly Lenore always calls me at six P.M. on my birthday and asks, "How does it feel to be a whole year older than you were yesterday?" Well, maybe I won't answer. I don't have to. I can go right on walking across the casino. . . .

No, I can't. It's all ruined. I don't even see him anymore, or Monte Carlo, either. I guess I'd better talk to Cousin Molly Lenore. She'll just keep calling until I do.

Oh, but maybe Someday I won't be here to answer, because I really *will* be dancing around a plaza in Mexico City or learning to blow glass in Venice or picking wildflowers on a Greek mountain. Someday.

Mixed Readings

PURPOSE

You are now able to maintain your practice pitch and proper tone focus on the short sentences. Some of the problems have been corrected, and midsection breathing should be in the process of becoming a life-style. What is needed at this level is practice, practice, practice. The more you concentrate on coordinating pitch, tone focus, and midsection breathing, the faster your voice skills will become automatic. Greater vocal variety can then be developed. The following selections begin to introduce volume, balanced resonance, and rate, which are also important aspects to be considered in the well-used voice. They have been carefully chosen for the increasing demands they place on your ability.

GOAL To maintain your practice pitch level and correct tone focus combined with the other vocal variables of volume, balanced resonance, and midsection breathing throughout short selections and paragraphs.

PROCEDURE

1. If needed, use the carrier phrase "hi" at the beginning of each selection to establish your correct pitch and tone focus.

2. Read each selection with as much vocal variety as possible and begin to coordinate midsection breath support.

3. A suggested way to integrate the vocal variables of pitch, tone focus, and breath support is to read each short paragraph three times. The first time you read the selection, think only of pitch and tone focus; the main goal for the second reading is midsection breath support; during the third reading you can try to combine pitch, tone focus, and midsection breathing into a total process.

4. Often the pitch drops toward the end of a longer reading and the proper tone focus is sometimes lost. Your awareness of this problem will help you to work harder at maintaining these two vocal variables throughout the entire reading.

EPITAPHS

Often when reading an epitaph, the mood will change to one of solemnity; the pitch of the voice usually drops into the lower register and the rate slows down. However, these epitaphs are different and may produce a lighter mood.

> The dust of Melantha Gribbling
> Swept up at last
> By the
> Great housekeeper

Stranger, tread
This ground with gravity:
Dentist Brown is filling
His last cavity

Here lies Pecos Bill
He always lied
And always will:
He once lied loud
He now lies still

Here lies the body
Of May Gwynne
Who was so very
Pure within
She cracked the shell
Of her earthly skin
And hatched herself
A cherubim

Here lies the body
Of our dear Anna
Done to death
By a banana:
It wasn't the fruit
That dealt the blow
But the skin of the thing
That laid her low

Poor Martha Snell
Her's gone away
Her would if her could
But her couldn't stay:
Her had two swoln legs
And a baddish cough
But her legs it was
As carried her off

She lived with
Her husband
Fifty years
And died in the
Confident hope
Of a better life

Beneath this stone
A lump of clay
Lies Uncle Peter Daniels:
Too early in the
Month of May
He took off his
Winter flannels

Comic Epitaphs from the
Very Best Old Graveyards

PARAGRAPHS

The following paragraphs have been chosen for their subject matter, which offers the opportunity to put into practice different levels of volume, colorful phrasing, and varying rates. They start simply and become increasingly more complex.

1. Nothing in the world can take the place of persistence. Talent will not; nothing is more common than unsuccessful men with talent. Genius will not; unrewarded genius is almost a proverb. Education alone will not; the world is full of educated derelicts. Persistence and determination alone are omnipotent.

Anonymous

2. Belief in something without personal experience and verification of facts is of little value. Modern man wants a well-defined and clear cut science which gives concrete results. We should see with our own eyes and hear with our own ears.

Kirpal Singh

3. The screech owls' dismal scream...is a most solemn graveyard ditty...Wise midnight hags! Yet I love to hear their wailing trilled along the woodside, as if it were the dark and tearful side of music, the regrets and sighs that would fain be sung.

Thoreau

4. A man's true greatness lies in the consciousness of an honest purpose in life, founded on a just estimate of himself and everything else, on frequent self-examinations, and a steady obedience to the rule which he knows to be right,

without troubling himself about what others may think or say, or whether they do or do not do that which he thinks and says and does.

Marcus Aurelius

5. To everything there is a season, and a time to every purpose under the heaven: a time to be born, and a time to die; a time to plant, and a time to pluck up that which has been planted; a time to kill, and a time to heal; a time to break down, and a time to build up; a time to weep, and a time to laugh; a time to mourn, and a time to dance; a time to cast away stones, and a time to gather stones together; a time to embrace, and a time to refrain from embracing; a time to get, and a time to lose; a time to keep, and a time to cast away; a time to rend and a time to sow; a time to keep silence and a time to speak; a time to love and a time to hate; a time of war, and a time of peace.

Ecclesiastes

6. Man is separated from the shark by an abyss of time. The fish still lives in the late Mesozoic, when the rocks were made: it has changed but little in perhaps three hundred million years. Across the gulf of ages, which evolved other marine creatures, the relentless, indestructible shark has come without need of evolution, the oldest killer, armed for the fray of existence in the beginning.

Jacques-Yves Cousteau
and James Dugan

7. Alice opened the door and found that it led into a small passage into the loveliest garden you ever saw. How she longed to get out of that dark hall, and wander among those beds of bright flowers and those cool fountains but she could not even get her head through the doorway: "It would be of little use even if my head *would* go through because my shoulders could not get through. Oh, how I wish I could shut up like a telescope! I think I could if I only knew how to begin." For, you see, so many out-of-the-way things had happened lately, that Alice had begun to think that nothing was impossible.

Lewis Carroll

8. And now was acknowledged the presence of the Red Death. He had come like a thief in the night. And one by one dropped the revelers in the blood-bedewed halls of their revel, and died each in the despairing posture of his fall. And the life of the ebony clock went out with that of the last of the gay. And the flames of the tripods expired. And Darkness and Decay and the Red Death held illimitable dominion over all.

Edgar Allan Poe

9. He was a popular man, but he had criticized the San Francisco authorities, among other things, and the welcome mat was wearing thin. A friend offered him refuge at the mountain retreat on Jackass Hill. Even in the mid-1860s this was not the liveliest spot in California, so our critic in hiding would amble into nearby Angels Camp and trade stories

with the miners. Story telling, the wilder the better, was his claim to fame. But nothing compared to what was about to happen. He heard a great story about a rigged frog jumping contest. He liked it, and from this story created what became one of the best known stories of the frontier, "The Celebrated Jumping Frog of Calaveras County." As soon as it was published, his fame spread from coast to coast. To this day, during the third week in May, Angels Camp holds a frog jumping jubilee in memory of the critic in hiding... Mark Twain.

from California Vignettes

10. I was directed at last to a very neat little cottage with cheerful bow windows, where a muslin curtain partly undrawn in the middle, a large round green screen or fan fastened onto the window sill, a small table, and a great chair suggested that my aunt might be seated there in awful state.

My shoes were by this time in a woeful condition. My shirt and trousers, stained with heat, dew, grass, and Kentish soil — and torn besides — might have frightened the birds from my aunt's garden. My hair had known no comb or brush since I left London. From head to foot I was powdered almost as white with chalk and dust as if I had come out of a lime kiln. In this plight I waited to make my first impression on my formidable aunt.

Charles Dickens

11. During the whole of a dull, dark, and soundless day in autumn of the year, when the clouds hung oppressively low in the heavens, I had been passing alone, on horseback,

through a singularly dreary tract of country; and at length found myself, as the shades of the evening drew on, within view of the melancholy House of Usher. I know not how it was—but, with the first glimpse of the building, a sense of gloom pervaded my spirit.

Edgar Allan Poe

12. Dream delivers us to dream, and there is no end to illusion. Life is a train of moods like a string of beads, and, as we pass through them, they prove to be many-colored lenses which paint the world their own hue, and each shows only what lies in its focus. From the mountain you see the mountain. We animate what we can, and we see only what we animate. Nature and books belong to the eyes that see them. It depends on the mood of the man, whether he shall see the sunset or the fine poem. There are always sunsets, and there is always genius...

Ralph Waldo Emerson

13. In the distance, a great white mass lazily rose, and rising higher and higher, and disentangling itself from the azure, at last gleamed before our prow like a snowslide, new slid from the hills. Thus glistening for a moment, as slowly it subsided, and sank. Then once more arose, and silently gleamed. It seemed not a whale; and yet is this Moby Dick? thought Daggoo. Again the phantom went down, but on reappearing once more, with a stiletto-like cry that startled every man from his nod, the Negro yelled out—"There! there again!

there she breaches! right ahead! The White Whale, the White Whale!"

Herman Melville

14. Eagles are not kindly birds. Some are cowardly and cruel. But the ancient race of the northern mountains were the greatest of all birds; they were proud and strong and noble-hearted. They did not love goblins, or fear them. When they took any notice of them at all (which was seldom, for they did not eat such creatures), they swooped on them and drove them shrieking back to their caves, and stopped whatever wickedness they were doing. The goblins hated the eagles and feared them, but could not reach their lofty seats, or drive them from the mountains.

J.R.R. Tolkien

15. Good Heaven! what was that which sent the blood tingling to his heart and deprived him of his voice and of power to move! There — there — at the window — close before him — so close, that he could have almost touched him before he started back — with his eyes peering into the room and meeting his — there stood Fagin! And beside him, white with rage or fear, or both, were the scowling features of the very man who had accosted him in the inn yard.

It was but an instant, a glance, a flash, before his eyes; and they were gone. But they had recognized him, and he them; and their look was firmly impressed upon his memory. He stood transfixed for a moment; then, leaping from the window into the garden, called loudly for help.

Charles Dickens

16. In the patches of silver sand the clams were stuck upright in small clusters, their mouths gaping. Sometimes, perched between the shell's horny lips, there would be a tiny, pale ivory pea-crab, the frail, soft-shelled, degenerate creature that lived a parasitic life in the safety of the great shell's corrugated walls. It was interesting to set off the clam colony's burglar alarm. I drifted over a group of them until they lay below, gaping up at me, and then gently edged the handle of the butterfly net down and tapped on the shell. Immediately the shell snapped shut, the movement causing a small puff of white sand to swirl up like a tornado. As the currents of this shell's alarm slid through the water the rest of the colony felt them. In a moment the water was full of little whirls of sand, drifting and swirling about the shells, falling back to the sea-bed like silver dust.

Gerald Durrell

17. Well, then. At the end of the earth stands a high mountain; on the top of this mountain is a huge boulder, and out of the boulder flows a stream of clear water. At the opposite end of the earth is the heart of the world. Now each thing in the world has a heart, and the world itself has a great heart of its own. And the heart of the world keeps the clear stream ever in sight, gazing at it with insatiable longing and desire. But the heart of the world can make not even one step toward it, for the moment it stirs from its place, it loses sight of the mountain's summit and the crystal spring. And if, though for a single instant only, it loses sight of the spring,

it loses in that same moment its life, and the heart of the world begins to die.

A. Ansky
(Solomon Rappoport)

18. The natural measure of this power is the resistance of circumstances. Impure men consider life as it is reflected in opinions, events and persons. They cannot see the action, until it is done. Yet its moral element pre-existed in the actor, and its quality as right or wrong, it was easy to predict. Everything in nature is bipolar, or has a positive and negative pole. There is a male and a female, a spirit and a fact, a north and a south. Spirit is the positive, the event is the negative. Will is the north, action the south pole. Character may be ranked as having its natural place in the north. It shares the magnetic currents of the system. The feeble souls are drawn to the south or negative pole. They look at the profit or hurt of the action. They never behold a principle until it is lodged in a person. They do not wish to be lovely, but to be loved...

Ralph Waldo Emerson

19. The star disappeared and the footsteps that accompanied it clanked out of hearing in the distance. Mr. Wright held up his lantern and the vague vastness took something of form itself — the stately columns developed stronger outlines, and a dim pallor here and there marked the places of lofty windows. We were among the tombs; and on every hand dull shapes of men, sitting, standing or stooping, inspected us curiously out of the darkness — reached out their

hands toward us—some appealing, some beckoning, some warning us away. Effigies, they were—statues over the graves; but they looked human and natural in the murky shadows. Now a little half-grown black-and-white cat squeezed herself through the bars of the iron gate and came purring lovingly about us, unawed by the time or the place—unimpressed by the marble pomp that sepulchers a line of mighty dead that ends with an author of yesterday and began with a sceptered monarch away back in the dawn of history more than twelve hundred years ago.

Mark Twain

20. Five minutes ago, Hareton seemed a personification of my youth, not a human being: I felt to him in such a variety of ways, that it would have been impossible to have accosted him rationally. In the first place, his startling likeness to Catherine connected him fearfully with her. That, however, which you may suppose the most potent to arrest my imagination, is actually the least: for what is not connected with her to me? and what does not recall her? I cannot look down to this floor, but her features are shaped in the flags! In every cloud, in every tree—filling the air at night, and caught by glimpses in every object by day—I am surrounded by her image! The most ordinary faces of men and women—my own features—mock me with a resemblance. The entire world is a dreadful collection of memoranda that she did exist, and that I have lost her!

Emily Brontë

21. He could now examine the panther at ease; its muzzle was smeared with blood . . .

It was a female. The fur on her belly and flanks was glistening white; many small marks like velvet formed beautiful bracelets around her feet; her sinuous tail was also white, ending with black rings; the overpart of her dress, yellow like unburnished gold, very lissom and soft, had the characteristic blotches in the form of rosettes, which distinguish the panther from every other feline species.

This tranquil and formidable hostess snored in an attitude as graceful as that of a cat lying on a cushion. Her blood-stained paws, nervous and well-armed, were stretched out before her face, which rested upon them, and from which radiated her straight, slender whiskers, like threads of silver.

Honoré de Balzac

22. During the night the seas piled up and became really fierce. Often it was quite uncanny to stand on the creaking, swaying steering bridge and see nothing in the world but a lighted patch of sail and the lamp at the masthead, which swung like an unruly moon among the stars when one glimpsed their light between racing storm clouds. Now and then a venomous snake seemed to be hissing right at one's back and a foaming wave crest would come rushing along at the height of one's head, invisible in its blackness apart from the white foam on top that seemed to be sailing along through the air, whispering to itself. The pursuing creature reached us and lifted us in the air with its huge watery muscles, only to let us go again and drop us so deep that the next white phantom following behind hovered over us at

a still greater height. We were worn out, dead tired, after two hour's intensive night watch at the two rudder-oars, even though we were generally using only one of them, allowing the other to work in a fixed position.

Thor Heyerdahl

POETRY

Poetry supports the speaker in the same way that music supports the dancer. As you read the poetry on the following pages, try to be aware of the rhythm and the way in which your voice not only enhances the words, but brings out the thoughts behind the words.

Black Africa

To become a chief's favorite
Is not always comfortable
It is like making friends
With a hippopotamus

Song of an Unlucky Man

Chaff is in my eye,
A crocodile has me by the leg,
A goat is in the garden,
A porcupine is cooking in the pot,
Meal is drying on the pounding rock,
The King has summoned me to court,
And I must go to the funeral of
my mother-in-law:
In short, I am busy

from A Crocodile
Has Me by the Leg

The day we die
Then the wind comes
To wipe us out,
The traces of our feet.

The wind creates dust
Which covers
The traces that were
Where we had walked,
For otherwise
It would be
As if we were
Still alive.
That is why it is the wind
That comes
To wipe out
The traces of our feet.

African bushman
(from Kalahari)

Dance of the Animals

I throw myself to the left,
I turn myself to the right,
I am the fish
Who glides in the water, who glides,
Who twists himself, who leaps.
Everything lives, everything dances, everything sings.

The bird flies,
Flies, flies, flies,
Goes, comes back, passes,
Mounts, hovers, and drops down.
I am the bird.
Everything lives, everything dances, everything sings.

The monkey, from bough to bough,
Runs, leaps, and jumps,
With his wife, with his little one,
His mouth full, his tail in the air:
This is the monkey, this is the monkey.
Everything lives, everything dances, everything sings.

Pygmy (from The
African Saga)

Ancient Mexico

I coyote-hungry-for-wisdom I say:
we are only a little while here
not forever on earth not forever on earth
only a little while
　　though it is jade it will be broken
　　though it is gold it will be crushed
　　though it is quetzal feather
　　it will be torn apart
not forever on earth not forever on earth
only a little while

*　*　*　*　*

Who will know my name?
　　at least my songs?
　　at least my flowers?
what is there to do?
are we here on earth for nothing?
　　at least my songs
　　at least my flowers

Nahautl (from 2-Rabbit
7-Wind: Poems from
Ancient Mexico)

CHINESE POEMS

Seeing You Off

Because you are seventy years old and
leaving, my handkerchief is wet with
tears . . . Because you are seventy years
old and have no home.

I am uneasy as the wind rises and your boat
sails off . . . White-headed traveler among
white-headed waves.

Po Chu-i

The Poet and the Flood

Icy winds sweep down from the mountains
and rip out the trees. Pitiless, the flood
rises in the river day by day. There is no
mountain now, or fields . . . everything is
fog and water.

All the same, my late chrysanthemums
are in bloom. When you row past, Yung-Hi,
slow your boat in front of my garden and gaze
at them . . . Their hot colors will rewarm
your heart.

Tu Fu

Eternity

The heaven endures forever and the Earth
is eternal. Why are Heaven and Earth

enduring and eternal? Because they do not live for themselves ... Therefore they can live forever.

The wise man desires to be forgotten, but he is remembered. He desires to be free of life, but he retains it. He desires nothing for himself, but he finds everything he wants.

from The Way of Virtue

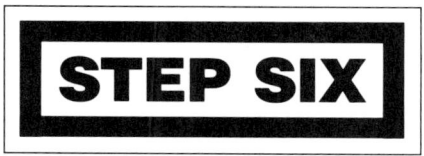

Long Selections

PURPOSE

By now your practice pitch and correct tone focus should be easier to produce. Continue to use this practice pitch on these longer readings to develop greater vocal strength. When your clinician thinks you are ready, you may begin reading at your optimal level. Midsection breathing should also be easier to accomplish. As you read longer selections, the next step is to make efforts to coordinate all of the vocal characteristics that you have been working on. The purpose, of course, is to maintain your new voice in an effortless way throughout the entire selection. At first you may find this is difficult. That's all right. Just keep practicing and you will discover that your voice will become stronger, and you will read these selections as smoothly as you now read the shorter ones.

The following selections have been carefully chosen with the phrasing and language in mind. The more sophisticated the language, the more skilled one must be in the use of the voice. When long selections can be read aloud easily with no vocal fatigue, a skill that places great demands on the voice has been mastered. Your practice will help you read these selections with greater ease, and you will begin to know what it is to have a voice that works for you under all circumstances. From this point it is a very short step toward carrying over your new voice into spontaneous conversation, which, of course, is the ultimate goal.

GOAL To coordinate all of the vocal variables: pitch, tone focus, quality, volume, rate, and breath support.

PROCEDURE

1. As you read the first two or three selections, use the carrier phrase "hi" at the beginning, in the middle, and at the end of the reading. The use of the carrier phrase is simply an aid to get you back on your pitch if it has begun to slip.

2. Midsection breath support and phrasing are especially important at this point.

3. Read some of the selections quietly and some with projection. You will find that certain selections lend themselves nicely to the element of volume.

4. As you become more confident in integrating the total vocal process, drop the carrier phrase and practice reading the selections in a natural way.

5. You may now read the selections in any order you wish.

6. Use your tape recorder for evaluating your voice objectively. Remember to tape-record and listen, tape-record and listen. This is necessary to fuse your subjective judgment with your objective judgment of what your voice really sounds like.

LONG SELECTIONS

1. St. Joseph's Day, March 19, finds thousands of visitors at the Mission San Juan Capistrano, awaiting the traditional arrival of the swallows. For on this date, for more than 180 years, flocks of swallows come home to the mission to nest and raise their young. Their punctuality is unvarying and unexplained . . . March 19 is "Swallow Day," even in a leap year.

Earlier, "scout" swallows will come to look things over, then evidently return to convoy the main flock. On arrival, the birds busy themselves by chasing out winter-resident sparrows and renewing their mud-and-grass nests on the mission's stone walls. Here they will stay until time for their winter trip south. As punctually as they arrive, the swallows leave each year by St. John's Day, October 23.

While "las golodrinas" as the Spanish call the swallows, are a great attraction, San Juan Capistrano itself has been called the Jewel of the Missions. Its great stone church, completed in 1806 and wrecked by earthquake in 1812, remains in ruins. Other, older buildings of the mission, founded in 1776, still stand as among California's oldest structures. Partial restoration of the Mission of the Swallows, in its setting of lovely gardens, perpetuates a bit of old Spanish California.

from California Vignettes

2. Can you imagine a stretch of grassy land bubbling like water in a pot? For that is really the best description of what was happening. In all directions it was swelling into humps. They were of very different sizes, some no bigger than mole-

hills, some as big as wheelbarrows, two the size of cottages. And the humps moved and swelled till they burst, and the crumbled earth poured out of them, and from each hump there came out an animal. The moles came out just as you might see a mole come out in England. The dogs came out, barking the moment their heads were free, and struggling as you've seen them do when they are getting through a narrow hole in a hedge. The stags were the queerest to watch, for of course the antlers came up a long time before the rest of them, so at first Digory thought they were trees. The frogs, who all came up near the river, went straight into it with a plop-plop and a loud croaking. The panthers, leopards, and things of that sort sat down at once to wash the loose earth off their hind quarters and then stood up against the trees to sharpen their front claws. Showers of birds came out of the trees. Butterflies fluttered. Bees got to work on the flowers as if they hadn't a second to lose. But the greatest moment of all was when the biggest hump broke like a small earthquake and out came the sloping back, the large, wise head, and the four baggy-trousered legs of an Elephant. And now you could hardly hear the song of the Lion; there was so much cawing, cooing, crowing, braying, neighing, baying, barking, lowing, bleating, and trumpeting.

C.S. Lewis (from The Magician's Nephew)

3. In a few minutes more, there came over the scene another radical alteration. The general surface grew somewhat more smooth, and the whirlpools, one by one, disappeared, while prodigious streaks of foam became apparent where none had

been seen before. These streaks, at length, spreading out to a greater distance and entering into combination, took unto themselves the gyratory motion of the subsided vortices, and seemed to form the germ of another more vast. Suddenly — very suddenly — this assumed a distinct and definite existence, in a circle of more than a mile in diameter. The edge of the whirl was represented by a broad belt of gleaming spray; but no particle of this slipped into the mouth of the terrific funnel, whose interior, as far as the eye could fathom it, was a smooth, shining, and jet-black wall of water, inclined to the horizon at an angle of some forty-five degrees, speeding dizzily round and round with a swaying and sweltering motion, and sending forth to the winds an appealing voice, half shriek, half roar, such as not even the mighty cataract of Niagara ever lifts up in its agony to Heaven.

Edgar Allan Poe (from A Descent into the Maelstrom)

4. Shortly Tom came upon the juvenile pariah of the village, Huckleberry Finn, son of the town drunkard. Huckleberry was cordially hated and dreaded by all the mothers of the town, because he was idle and lawless and vulgar and bad — and because all their children admired him so, and delighted in his forbidden society, and wished they dared to be like him. Tom was like the rest of the respectable boys, in that he envied Huckleberry his gaudy outcast condition, and was under strict orders not to play with him. So he played with him every time he got a chance. Huckleberry was always dressed in the cast-off clothes of full-grown men, and they were in perennial bloom and fluttering with rags. His hat

was a vast ruin with a wide crescent lopped out of its brim; his coat, when he wore one, hung nearly down the back; but one suspender supported his trousers; the seat of the trousers bagged low and contained nothing; the fringed legs dragged in the dirt when not rolled up.

Huckleberry came and went, at his own free will. He slept on door-steps in fine weather and in empty hogsheads in wet; he did not have to go to school or to church, or call any being master or obey anybody; he could go fishing or swimming when and where he chose, and stay as long as it suited him; nobody forbade him to fight; he could sit up as late as he pleased; he was always the first boy that went barefoot in the spring and the last to resume leather in the fall; he never had to wash, nor put on clean clothes; he could swear wonderfully. In a word, everything that goes to make life precious that boy had. So thought every harassed, hampered, respectable boy in St. Petersburg.

Mark Twain (from
Tom Sawyer)

5. For a week or so the wind played with the island, patting it, stroking it, humming to itself among the bare branches. Then there was a lull, a few days' strange calm; suddenly, when you least expected it, the wind would be back. But it was a changed wind, a mad, hooting, bellowing wind that leaped down on the island and tried to blow it into the sea. The blue sky vanished as a cloak of fine grey cloud was thrown over the island. The sea turned a deep blue, almost black, and became crusted with foam. The cypress trees were whipped like dark pendulums against the sky, and the

olives (so fossilized all summer, so still and witchlike) were infected with the madness of the wind and swayed creaking on their misshapen, sinewy trunks, their leaves hissing as they turned, like mother of pearl, from green to silver. This is what the dead leaves had whispered about, this is what they had practiced for; exultantly they rose in the air and danced, whirligigging about, dipping, swooping, falling exhausted when the wind tired of them and passed on. Rain followed the wind, but it was a warm rain that you could walk in and enjoy, great fat drops that rattled on the shutters, tapped on the vine leaves like drums, and gurgled musically in the gutters. The rivers up in the Albanian mountains became swollen and showed white teeth in a snarl as they rushed down to the sea, tearing at their banks, grabbing the summer debris of sticks, logs, grass tussocks, and other things and disgorging them into the bay, so that the dark-blue waters became patterned with great coiling veins of mud and other flotsam. Gradually all these veins burst, and the sea changed from blue to yellow-brown; then the wind tore at the surface, piling the water into ponderous waves, like great tawny lions with white manes that stalked and leaped upon the shore.

Gerald Durrell (from My Family and Other Animals)

6. If it wasn't for Chewing Gum, Americans would wear their teeth off just hitting them against each other. Every Scientist has been figuring out who the different races descend from. I don't know about the other tribes, but I do know that the American Race descended from the Cow. And Wrigley was

smart enough to furnish the Cud. He has made the whole World chew for Democracy.

That's why this subject touches me so deeply. I have chewed more Gum than any living Man. My Act on the Stage depended on the grade of Gum I chewed. Lots of my readers have seen me and perhaps noted the poor quality of my jokes on that particular night. Now I was not personally responsible for that. I just happened to hit on a poor piece of Gum. One can't always go by the brand. There just may be a poor stick of Gum in what otherwise may be a perfect package. It may look like the others on the outside but after you get warmed up on it, why, you will find that it has a flaw in it. And hence my act would suffer. I have always maintained that big Manufacturers of America's greatest necessity should have a Taster—a man who personally tries every Piece of Gum put out.

Now lots of People don't figure the lasting quality of Gum. I have had Gum that wouldn't last you over half a day, while there are others which are like Wine—they improve with Age.

I had a certain piece of Gum once, which I used to park on the Mirror of my dressing room after each show. Why, you don't know what a pleasure it was to chew that Gum. It had a kick, or spring to it, that you don't find once in a thousand Packages. I have always thought it must have been made for Wrigley himself.

And say, what jokes I thought of while chewing that Gum! Ziegfeld himself couldn't understand what had put such life and Humor into my Work.

Then one night it was stolen, and another piece was substituted in its place, but the minute I started in to work on this other Piece I knew that someone had made a switch. I knew this was a Fake. I hadn't been out on the Stage 3 minutes until half the audience were asleep and the other half were hissing me. So I just want to say you can't exercise too much care and judgement in the selection of your Gum, because if it acts that way with me in my work, it must do the same with others, only they have not made the study of it that I have. . . .

Now, some Gum won't stick easy. It's hard to transfer from your hand to the Chair. Other kinds are heavy and pull hard. It's almost impossible to remove them from Wood or Varnish without losing a certain amount of the Body of the Gum.

There is lots to be said for Gum. This pet Piece of mine I afterwards learned had been stolen by a Follies Show Girl, who two weeks later married an Oil Millionaire.

> *Will Rogers (from* A Prospectus for the Remodeled Chewing Gum Corporation*)*

7. The prodigious strain upon the main-sail had parted the weather-sheet, and the tremendous boom was flying from side to side, completely sweeping the entire after part of the deck. The poor fellow whom Queequeg had handled so roughly, was swept overboard; all hands were in a panic; and to attempt snatching at the boom to stay it, seemed madness. It flew from right to left, and back again, almost in one ticking of a watch, and every instant seemed on the point of snapping into splinters. Nothing was done, and nothing

seemed capable of being done; those on deck rushed towards the bows, and stood eyeing the boom as if it were the lower jaw of an exasperated whale. In the midst of this consternation, Queequeg dropped deftly to his knees, and crawling under the patch of the boom, whipped hold of a rope, secured one end to the bulwarks, and then flinging the other like a lasso, caught it round the boom as it swept over his head, and at the next jerk, the spar was that way trapped, and all was safe. The schooner was run into the wind, and while the hands were clearing away the stern boat, Queequeg, stripped to the waist, darted from the side with a long living arc of a leap. For three minutes or more he was seen swimming like a dog, throwing his long arms straight out before him, and by turns revealing his brawny shoulders through the freezing foam. I looked at the grand and glorious fellow, but saw no one to be saved. The greenhorn had gone down. Shooting himself perpendicularly from the water, Queequeg now took an instant's glance around him, and seeming to see just how matters were, dived down and disappeared. A few minutes more, and he rose again, one arm still striking out, and with the other dragging a lifeless form. The boat soon picked them up. The poor bumpkin was restored. All hands voted Queequeg a noble trump; the Captain begged his pardon. From that hour I clove to Queequeg like a barnacle; yea, till poor Queequeg took his last long dive.

Herman Melville
(from Moby Dick)

8. On the first morning of the first rehearsal of the play, we were all gathered on stage at the old Mesa Theater in

Los Angeles waiting for the arrival of our star, Sir Francis Curran. This honored player was reputed to be only one rung down the theatrical ladder from Lord Laurence Olivier, who was, some maintained, himself sharing a rung with God.

While our director had actually met Sir Francis, the rest of us had only glimpsed him on stage (that is, if we'd been in London when he was performing) or in the few movies he had made in his twenty-six-year career. Sir Francis wasn't old; he just seemed that way, probably because at the age of twenty-eight, he had played Disraeli, soon following that with Oliver Cromwell, Martin Luther, Saint Paul, Copernicus, Pope Urban II, and King Lear.

Then, at thirty-five, he had become quite ancient with his portrayal of Merlin the Magician, topped off by a BBC-TV special in which he appeared as Methuselah.

I don't know what we expected that morning — perhaps a doddering forty-six-year-old, barely able to make it to the stage, supported by male nurses, oxygen tank and personal physician. Instead, one of the aisle doors opened (Sir Francis had not used the stage entrance) and down this carpeted path walked a small, slight individual, trailed by an equally diminutive valet. The actor wore a suit the color of London in February, reminding me of Lady Ann Sadler's remark years ago when she first saw him: "Who is that grey little shadow in the corner?"

He was reputed to be shy, and I must say that morning I thought he had every reason to be, for he resembled nothing so much as an aging bellhop; thinning hair, sunless face, with a kind of resigned expectancy, as if knowing he'd be summoned at any moment by a desk clerk.

We watched him greet our director (an effusive Austrian) who grandly escorted him up the steps and onto the stage to introduce him to the rest of us.

In this interim something happened. Though at close range the actor's pale, weary face seemed as vulnerable as a child's, when he looked at each of us in turn, his expression sharpened as if forming instant, irrevocable impressions, and then the man smiled. "I'm so pleased to meet all of you," he said quietly in a voice like an ebony cello. Its sound caused the backs of my knees to prickle, for soft as it was, it touched every pore of my skin, the threads of the curtains, the splinters in the floor. And his smile transformed him into a gentle, piquant sage who saw us all, accepted us all, and if the time ever came, would forgive us all.

I had a feeling this might turn out to be quite a play.

C. Garcia (from The Play)

9. Damon was one of those people I always wished I could get to know, though I'm sure he had little desire to know me. From the age of two until he left for college, he lived across the street, and I spoke to the boy only briefly on the occasions we did run into each other: usually our conversations concerned animals, such as my giant dog, Asa, in whom he showed an affectionate, if guarded, interest.

Damon reminded me of my long dead father, not so much in appearance, though both were dark haired and small boned for males, but in his carriage, his thoughtful speech, and in the way he seemed to value solitude. Damon got on well with other children, but he was never one of them, did not seek their approval, nor was he swayed by their values or behavior. His thin, serious face just missed severity due to the size of his eyes, which were over-large and green, and quiet as ponds on some vast estate.

One afternoon when he was about eleven, a group of young neighborhood stalwarts were engaged in a contest to see how far they could all spit. Some achieved an amazing distance of several feet, their scores being measured by a pigtailed female in a sweatshirt who was anxious to be accepted as one of them, and willing to act as a toady for the privilege. When Damon's turn came, she barked out his name in the manner of a pompous subordinate so that her broken front tooth was particularly prominent. I don't believe he had quite realized his role in this street scene until her voice jarred him out of a daydream, and he appeared startled, then a bit saddened. Again the female barked, "Damon, spit!" stirring him to action. I saw him step away from the group. "No," he said. "My mother wouldn't like it."

"Your mother's dead," one of the fellows reminded him.

"She still wouldn't like it," he replied and walked off down the street.

I remember, I used to see him sitting in the movies quite alone (as was I), his green eyes gazing intently up at the screen, chewing popcorn without a sound. Once I invited Damon and several of his acquaintances into the backyard to see my black and red Japanese salamander, which impressed them enough to prompt all sorts of questions, such as "Will he bite?" "Does he eat worms?" "How can he breathe under water?" I noted that Damon was the only child who asked about the health and longevity of such creatures in captivity.

Last fall he went away to the university, and I've missed him as I still miss my father and all the people in my life whom I found more fascinating or mysterious or lovable than they found me. Ah, well. Summer vacation is almost upon us. If Damon doesn't take a freighter to Morocco or Istanbul or Bombay, perhaps by this time next week, he will have come home again.

Damon *by C. Garcia*

10. This exercise is specifically for those of you who are interested in additional work on volume, phrasing, and breath control.

Ladies and gentlemen, boys and girls, oldsters, youngsters: Welcome to you all. Can you see me clearly? Does each and every one of you have an unobstructed view? I have here in my hand a small glass cask, a phial, a bottle, if you will, of Dr. Dankley's famous rejuvenating and miracle restorer. Just a drop or two of this amazing elixir in your coffee, tea, sarsaparilla, or even — for the more worldly — a glass of gooseberry wine. Yes, a few drops of this unique liquid will perform wonders before your eyes and the eyes of your loved ones. Now be honest, ladies and gentlemen, be truthful with yourselves. Are you victimized by occasional or possibly frequent attacks of insomnia, breathlessness, hiccups, migraine, canker sores, belching, eyestrain, fever blisters, liver spots, sneezing, gasping, fainting, or hysterical bursts into song? If you suffer from any or all of these grievous symptoms, even on the rarest occasions, your health, indeed, your entire well being, cannot be considered out of danger until you've placed a bottle of Dr. Dankley's rejuvenating and miracle restorer on the shelf of your medicine cabinet. Think of it, ladies and gentlemen, consider what I say . . . What's that, young fellow? You ask how does the elixir perform these diverse services? I'm so pleased you spoke up; I certainly am, for I find nothing more invigorating than to be in the presence of an inquiring mind . . . well, my youthful friend, I will explain how this astonishing product works, and it works in many and varied ways, its wonders to perform.

Among other things, Dr. Dankley's rejuvenating and miracle restorer *talks* to the body — yes, it actually sets up a sympathetic dialogue with the poor, afflicted area. For instance, it soothes the spleen, it flatters the pancreas, it praises the pituitary, it calms the bladder, it pampers the kidneys, it cajoles the colon, it encourages the sphincters, it coaxes the corneas, it compliments the bile, it humors the capillaries, it applauds the medulla oblongata — and it always, always titillates the taste buds.

Ladies and gentlemen, I heartily urge you not to delay by so much as a single moment in your purchase of this rare and marvelous curative. Why, in the last charming hamlet I visited, only one man — the venerable schoolmaster — demurred, and I am devastated to report, was buried the following Monday. So, step right up, my good friends, please do not dally. Who will be the first to take home a guarantee of radiant, lifelong health? I have it right here in my hand, ladies and gentlemen, right here! — Dr. Dankley's famous rejuvenating and miracle restorer.

C. *Garcia*

11. Our solid American citizen awakens in a bed built on a pattern which originated in the Near East but which was modified in Northern Europe before it was transmitted to America. He throws back covers made from cotton, domesticated in India, or linen, domesticated in the Near East, or wool from sheep, also domesticated in the Near East, or silk, the use of which was discovered in China. All of these materials have been spun and woven by processes invented in the Near East. He slips into his moccasins, invented by the Indians of the Eastern Woodlands, and goes to the bathroom, whose fixtures are a mixture of European and American inventions, both of recent date. He takes off his pajamas, a garment invented in India, and washes with soap invented by the ancient Gauls. He then shaves, a masochistic rite which seems to have been derived from either Sumer or ancient Egypt.

Returning to the bedroom, he removes his clothes from a chair of southern European type and proceeds to dress. He puts on garments whose form originally derived from the skin clothing of the nomads of the Asiatic steppes, puts on shoes made from skins tanned by a process invented in ancient Egypt and cut to a pattern derived from the classical civilizations of the Mediterranean, and ties around his neck a strip of bright-colored cloth which is a vestigial survival of the shoulder shawls worn by the seventeenth-century Croatians. Before going out for breakfast he glances through the window, made of glass invented in Egypt, and if it is raining puts on overshoes made of rubber discovered by the Central American Indians and takes an umbrella, invented in South-eastern Asia. Upon his head he puts a hat made of felt, a material invented in the Asiatic steppes.

On his way to breakfast he stops to buy a paper, paying for it with coins, an ancient Lydian invention. At the restaurant a whole new series of borrowed elements confronts him. His plate is made of a form of pottery invented in China. His knife is of steel, an alloy first made in southern India, his fork a medieval *Italian* invention, and his spoon a derivative of a Roman original. He begins breakfast with an orange, from the eastern Mediterranean, a cantaloupe from *Persia*, or perhaps a piece of African watermelon. With this he has coffee, an Abyssinian plant, with cream and sugar. Both the domestication of cows and the idea of milking them originated in the Near East, while sugar was first made in India. After his fruit and first coffee he goes on to waffles, cakes made by a Scandinavian technique from wheat domesticated in Asia Minor. Over these he pours maple syrup, invented by the Indians of the Eastern Woodlands. As a side dish he may have the egg of a species of bird domesticated in Indo-China, or thin strips of the flesh of an animal domesticated in Eastern Asia which have been salted and smoked by a process developed in northern Europe.

When our friend has finished eating he settles back to smoke, an American Indian habit, consuming a plant domesticated in Brazil in either a pipe, derived from the Indians of Virginia, or a cigarette, derived from Mexico. If he is hardy enough he may even attempt a cigar, transmitted to us from the Antilles by way of Spain. While smoking he reads the news of the day, imprinted in characters invented by the ancient Semites upon a material invented in China by a process invented in Germany. As he absorbs the accounts of foreign troubles he will, if he is a good conservative citizen, thank a Hebrew deity in an Indo-European language that he is 100% AMERICAN!

Ralph Linton (from The American Case*)*

12. There isn't any reason
Why a sentence, I suppose, once it begins
Once it has risen to the lips at all
And finds itself happily wandering
Through shady vowels and over consonants
Where ink's been spilt like rivers or like blood
Flowing for the cause of some half-truth
Or a dogma now outmoded, shouldn't go
Endlessly moving in grave periphrasis
And phrase in linking phrase, with commas falling
As airily as lime flowers, intermittently,
Uninterrupting, scarcely troubling
The mild and fragile progress of the sense
Which trills trebling like a pebble stream
Or lowers towards an oath-intoning ocean
Or with a careless and forgetful music
Looping and threading, tuning and entwining,
Flings a babel of bells, a carolling
Of such various vowels the ear can almost feel
The soul of sound when it lay in chaos yearning
For the tongue to be created: such a hymn
If not as lovely, then as interminable,
As restless, and as heartless, as the hymn

Which in the tower of heaven the muted spheres
With every rippling harp and windy horn
Played for incidental harmony
Over the mouldering rafters of the world
Rafters which seldom care to ring, preferring
The functional death-watch beetle, stark, staccato,
Economical as a knuckle bone,
Strict, correct, but undelighting
Like a cleric jiggling in the saturnalia,
The saturnalia we all must keep,
Green-growing and rash with life,
Our milchy, mortal, auroral, jovial,
Harsh, unedifying world,
Where every circle of grass can show a dragon
And every pool's as populous as Penge,
Where birds, with taffeta flying, scarf the air
On autumn evenings, and a sentence once
Begun goes on and on, there being no reason
To draw to any conclusion so long as breath
Shall last, except that breath
Can't last much longer.

Christopher Fry (from
Venus Observed)

13. Go placidly amid the noise and haste, and remember what peace there may be in silence. As far as possible without surrender, be on good terms with all persons. Speak your truth quietly and clearly; and listen to others, even the dull and ignorant; they too have their story. Avoid loud and aggressive persons, they are vexations to the spirit. If you

compare yourself with others you may become vain and bitter; for always there will be greater and lesser persons than yourself. Enjoy your achievements as well as your plans. Keep interested in your own career, however humble, it is a real possession in the changing fortunes of time. Exercise caution in your business affairs; for the world is full of trickery. But let this not blind you to what virtue there is; many persons strive for high ideals; and everywhere life is full of heroism. Be yourself. Especially, do not feign affection. Neither be cynical about love; for in the face of all aridity and disenchantment it is perennial as the grass. Take kindly the counsel of the years, gracefully surrendering the things of youth. Nurture strength of spirit to shield you in sudden misfortune. But do not distress yourself with imaginings. Many fears are born of fatigue and loneliness. Beyond a wholesome discipline, be gentle with yourself. You are a child of the universe, no less than the trees and the stars; you have a right to be here. And whether or not it is clear to you, no doubt the universe is unfolding as it should. Therefore, be at peace with God, whatever you conceive him to be, and whatever your labors and aspirations, with your soul. With all its sham, drudgery and broken dreams, it is still a beautiful world. Be careful. Strive to be happy.

Desiderata

14. I myself was not overly fond of these tournaments, but to my master, Sir Percy of Frottle, they were truly auspicious events. Sir Percy aspired to the Round Table, but unless Arthur became senile someday, aspiration was the closest Sir Percy would ever get to the venerable hunk of wood.

I was sorry to think this about my master, but he was often a dolt, a stumbler, and a booby wit. Worse, I was always included in his sallies forth upon the playing fields of Camelot, for he galloped me up to the King's stand with the royal canopy flapping above it and the court ladies fluttering beneath it, I staggering under the weight of his armor and saddle, not to mention the lance that he gripped like a toddler does its mother's thumb.

On that particular day of which I now speak, a great contest had been announced and every knight in England had answered the call, each one signing up for a joust with an appropriate partner of equal skill and prowess. Unfortunately, nobody was in my master's class, and he was hard put, spending the morning roaming among the younger lads, even some servants, for a likely prospect. Alas, none was forthcoming. This shattered him, I knew, though he showed a brave face and did indeed keep his armor on, stomping and clanking about the ground, ripping up grass with his metal feet, lifting his vizor to wink at the ladies, who howled with laughter. Sir Percy grinned back at them, pretending it was a joke as he searched for a partner, though I knew his heart must have slipped way down toward his belly. Oh, Percy was a fool, but a sweet fool.

It was then I saw Queen Guinevere slip into Sir Lancelot's tent and I turned to see if Sir Percy had seen them, too; he had. Now, this romance was the scandal of the land, rumors of it even reaching the Italian and German kings; in fact, everyone but Arthur. We all knew it was only a matter of time until *he* got wind of it, too, probably through that viper, that kinsman of his, Sir Modred. Now, if Guinevere had been less beautiful or less kind, and if Lancelot had not been so brave, and if they had not been in agony because of their dangerous attraction, nobody would have given a pea what Modred said. But—suddenly I felt Sir Percy start and grasp my bridle. "It's Modred," he whispered.

Sure as a bellyache after a banquet, that asp was making his way toward Lancelot's tent, no doubt to eavesdrop; he had a memory like a parrot.

Without warning my master clambered and clanked into his saddle, making the most awful racket, his metal gloves grasping my neck and mane, his feet searching desperately for a stirrup. When seated he leaned down to my ear and said, "Let's get him."

To this day I don't know what possessed me. (My love for the Queen? My pity for Lancelot and Arthur? Sir Percy's misplaced toe in my left flank?) But I began turning and bucking and whinnying, all the while heading toward Modred, wondering if I could slip between him and the tent, and then drive him away from the place, and give the Queen a chance to escape.

By now the crowd was roaring at my antics and at Percy who was hanging on to me, bobbing like a pile of metal shingles, his armor scraping and screeching in a tinny symphony as I bucked and pranced over to Modred who had begun backing away. He looked like a mollusk of some sort, with his crab-like steps; I fairly pounded down upon him, and sent him scurrying across the jousting field, with Sir Percy and me in pursuit, the crowd cheering now (they detested the knave too), King Arthur's face puzzled but amused— suddenly I tripped in a gopher hole, righted myself, but sent

Sir Percy and his lance sprawling. There he lay in a clanking pile, flopping like a tortoise on its back. I leaned down in apology, but just then his vizor fell open and he winked at me. "Good work," he said. "I think we saved the Queen today."

I thought so too, and just to make sure, I cantered off down the field after the quick stepping schemer.

The Horse's Aspect
by C. Garcia

STEP SEVEN

Carryover Activities

PURPOSE

You are now approaching the last step in the process of vocal rehabilitation. Carryover of the new voice into spontaneous conversation is of course the ultimate goal. Using the voice spontaneously sometimes presents difficulties in that when we are engaged in a conversation our thoughts take over and the way we are expressing those thoughts is forgotten; therefore some practice is needed to bridge the gap between structured "exercises" and your spontaneous speech. The following carryover activities have been successful. You may think of others.

GOAL To use the new voice as a life-style.

PROCEDURE

1. Each suggested carryover activity is self-explanatory; however, with the "out of the clinical setting" suggestions you need to have a keen awareness of appropriate pitch and volume for each situation.

2. Try not to compete with the background noises by attempting to speak louder; speak under the noise. The surrounding noise is traveling through the air into your outer ear, psychologically creating an illusion that you have to speak louder. It's just the opposite. While maintaining your new voice, speak normally. You may think that you are barely being heard. This, too, is an illusion and you will find that by not competing with the noise, you are being heard clearly by your listener and no vocal strain is felt.

CARRYOVER ACTIVITIES

1. Telephone

When possible place the tape recorder near the phone. As you make a phone call or answer the phone, turn the tape recorder on in order to record the conversation. Listen immediately following the conversation to your recorded voice and make your judgments accordingly. "Did I maintain my pitch level?" "Was the volume too loud or too soft?" "Did I start the conversation using my new voice and then become involved in thought and fall back into my old ways?" or "I *did* use my voice effectively throughout the conversation." Several phone calls made in this way will help you to be more aware of the way you use your voice.

2. Magazines

Choose a magazine such as *National Geographic*. Select any picture you wish; read its caption as if it were an exercise. This helps to establish the vocal variables upon which you have been working. Move immediately away from the reading and begin to describe the picture using your own thoughts and words. Tape-record and listen back. Again judge your ability to maintain your new voice from the beginning of the exercise to the end.

3. Newspapers

Read any newspaper article as if it were a voice exercise. Then retell the article in your own words carrying over your newly acquired voice. Tape-record and listen.

4. Recall

Take a few minutes at the end of your day and begin to recall the major incidents of the day starting from the period after dinner and working back in time to your breakfast. Tape-record and listen. This exercise places demands upon your attention and your ability to remember your voice as well as the happenings of the day.

5. Conversations

Set aside 5 or 10 minutes a day during which you will have a conversation with a member of the family, a colleague, or a friend. The primary purpose of this conversation is to be aware of the way you are using your voice. True, you may have an awareness of your voice throughout the day, but often your memory goes in and out of a situation and you realize you have forgotten to listen to yourself speak. To select a goal that is more consciously chosen may improve your ability to remember to use your new voice while interacting with another person.

PROBLEMS IN PUBLIC PLACES

1. Speaking Outdoors

Any outdoor activity, such as walking on a busy street or sitting at the beach, presents situations that can be taxing on a voice. Outdoor sounds dissipate rapidly and again your judgment in the use of volume is inaccurate. Do not try to outdo the noise, but speak under it to be heard.

2. Eating in a Restaurant

Whenever you have the opportunity to eat in a restaurant, be aware of the background noises. The tendency may be to lower your pitch and increase your volume. Do the opposite; maintain your natural pitch and correct tone focus. Volume should be less than the background noises. Your listener will tell you if you cannot be heard, and experience will teach you the appropriate volume.

3. Riding in a Car

Riding in a car creates an atmosphere of tension when the voice is improperly used. You are having to cope with noise such as highway sounds, air conditioning, and radios, and often at the same time one's conversations need to be directed into the backseat while having to face forward. Any of these alone is enough to place demands upon the voice. Simply by being aware of these particular circumstances you can monitor your voice in a more efficient way.

Step by step you have moved from an inefficient voice to one that is healthy and spontaneous. The change has taken time, and practice has been the discipline that has brought you the fulfillment of your vocal goals, so enjoy the new experience and . . . **go jolly.**